Get Your RAW On

Get Your RAW On

Reach And Win your transition to a healthier you

Terri Eileen Liggins

The Literary Front Publishing Company
Las Vegas, Nevada

Published by The Literary Front Publishing Company
Las Vegas, Nevada

Cover design by The Literary Front
Typesetting services by bookow.com

Printed in the United States of America

ISBN 978-1-7366866-7-6
Library of Congress Control Number: 2025920882

For more information, visit: terriliggins.com

Dedication

I dedicate this book to all the open-minded people who instead of saying, "That could never happen," can muster up an ounce of hope to ask, "How can we make it happen?" Because...

It was open mindedness in 2000 that allowed me to seek a healthy alternative after a serious chronic illness diagnosis. (I knew there had to be a better way than my 15 different medications.)

It was open-mindedness in 2002 that allowed me to follow Bill and Joyce Frederick's anti-candida yeast diet after just meeting them and learning of Joyce's miraculous healing. (I don't believe in coincidences; our meeting was truly a divine encounter.)

It was open mindedness in 2012 that allowed me to listen to nutrition expert Chef Keidi Awadu's extensively researched findings on the dangers of some foods and healing attributes of other foods and soon ask, "How can I reach my healthiest state once and for all?"

Why do I strive for that pinnacle of optimum health? Because I'm here for a purpose beyond myself. To discover that purpose, I need to be the best me.

When I'm unhealthy in body and emotion, my mind says, "That could never happen." When I'm well in my body and sharp in my mind, my thoughts are fixed on, "How can we make this happen?" What is it I want to make happen? A better community. A better nation. A better planet.

To create a better planet, I as an individual and we as a nation must think sustainability. We must make greatness permanent. We must think environmentally-sound thoughts. We must bring forth positive improvements. We must accept that we are called here for a specific purpose bigger than ourselves; stretching further than our own lifetime.

But first, we must have the open mindedness to believe our healthiest self is necessary to successfully fulfill that purpose on this earth.

Be open-minded!

Foreword

As a physician, I see the faces every day of those who desire to regain their vibrant, healthy self but feel it is far out of their reach. That's when I'm most grateful for my role as a physician to be able to guide them to make healthier lifestyle choices as part of their treatment for a successful outcome.

I applaud Terri for writing this book, chronicling her personal journey toward that same desire of optimal health and vibrant longevity. Her book shows the reader how such a goal is not out of reach, but instead, right at their fingertips. Her testimony and knowledge about the barriers dealing with nutrition that one needs to overcome are spot on and will serve as a bright beacon for anyone else who is sick and tired of being sick and tired.

I work alongside a whole team of amazingly talented wellness experts at Cleveland Clinic, one of the top-ranked medical institutions in the nation. Even still, we rely on great chemistry and a solid doctor-patient relationship in improving patient outcomes—each one bringing their A-game to the table.

I love how *Get Your RAW On* encourages and empowers its readers to stay on top of their health. And should they happen to become a patient, they will be the most well-informed, A-game patient on the road to a quick recovery.

I appreciate Terri as a friend and have enjoyed working with her professionally. I look forward to other publications from her in the future.

Linda D. Bradley, MD, Cleveland Clinic

Co-Author of *Us! Our Life. Our Health. Our Legacy.* (2016)

Professor of Surgery

Vice Chair of the Obstetrics, Gynecology and Women's Health Institute Director of the

Fibroid and Menstrual Disorders Center

Director of Hysteroscopic Services

Disclaimer

In addition to researched and learned information, this book contains personal journal entries the author made during her first year of going "cold turkey" from a Standard American Diet (SAD) to raw, plant-based, living superfoods. As the experiences and opinions set forth in this book are her own, they are not intended as professional medical advice for you, the reader. Please consult a healthcare provider, nutritionist or other qualified professional for proper diagnosis and consultation before making changes to your diet and/or exercise routine. Also, you should never stop taking medication without first consulting the physician who prescribed it.

The author and publisher expressly disclaim all responsibility for any liability, loss or risk incurred as a result of using or applying any methods or preparing and consuming any foods shared in this book. Keep in mind that every person is unique. What may benefit 999,999 out of 1,000,000 people, may not benefit you at all.

In Memory

Parri Strickland Womack, ascended July 19, 2009 at age 51

Virginia Ann Earley, ascended March 23, 2011 at age 51

Juana Rene' Johnson, ascended September 25, 2013 at age 56

Charmaine Ali, ascended August 9, 2014 at age 60

Larry Carter, ascended September 21, 2014 at age 56

Five wonderful people. Whether a college mate, relative or BFF, all were in my life for long seasons and special reasons. They were all at or near my same age when they ascended into the heavenlies—too soon, too young. Their spirits will forever live in my heart.

It is in the spirit of these precious lives that I encourage others to live their life long and strong by believing and accepting the fact that there IS another way to handle diseases and illnesses. Don't leave it up to the fund-raising foundations. Instead, read what the scientists have been stating for years.

Close examination of those foundations will show their true colors. For instance, one well-known "pink" group has collected billions of dollars over 30 years to find a cure for cancer. Still no cure? Nonsense. Cancer cures have been out there since the 1930s. What, this foundation hasn't told you that? Why should they? That would only stop the flow of massive amounts of money you're running, walking and biking for to place in the pockets of administrators.

Stop the madness, people! *You* can reduce or reverse the pathogens causing cancer and other diseases. Read this book. Do your research. You got this!

Whether you dive in 100% and take your health back with a vengeance like I did, or you approach it in stages, just know that if you are given a dismal prognosis from your doctor, you DO NOT have to accept it! Don't you deserve to know that there IS an alternative to deadly drugs, radiation, chemotherapy and the carving up of your body? The alternative is through healthy lifestyle choices. If you're not able to make those choices on your own, hire a nutritionist or health coach.

Parri, Virginia, Juana, Charmaine, Larry and millions of other deceased cancer patients deserved to live disease free. Cancer patients today, fighting for their lives, deserve to live disease free. People fighting diabetes, cardiovascular and high blood pressure diseases, Alzheimer's, chronic auto immune and so many other issues, all deserve to live disease free. YOU deserve to live disease free. Claim that freedom today! This book will help you learn how.

Contents

Part I

My Why's

Chapter 1
My Testimony

Funny how RAW spelled backwards is WAR

Boy, was I at war when I first went raw! I didn't know I was inviting a war when I decided to start eating healthier, but I should've seen it coming. Anytime someone steps outside their comfort zone to make a change for the better—ridding excess weight, making more money and other forms of self-development —friction is bound to happen.

1. First of all, my flesh waged war against my spirit, telling me things like it should be okay to have just one slice of pizza, or just one more Protein Burger (that's a hamburger without the bun from the unpublicized menu of *In and Out Burger*) for old time's sake.

2. Secondly, my ego waged war against my intellect. It insisted that since I'm neither obese nor diagnosed with a life-threatening disease like cancer I'm a fairly healthy person who can just keep living life as is (as though sarcoidosis' fatality rate would never include me in its stats).

3. Finally, other people waged war against my character, belittling *me* as the bad guy. Yes, I'm the nuisance for sharing nutritional knowledge that will save lives; meanwhile, America's big food manufacturers, advertisers and government food agencies—who normalize junk foods, fast foods and processed foods for the sake of the almighty dollar—are heralded as having our best interest at heart. Go figure.

Terri Eileen Liggins

Here's what brought me to my current raw lifestyle

In November 1999, I suffered a heart attack.[1] I was just 40 and caught totally off guard. That incidence led to a battery of tests, scans and biopsies until a diagnosis of a serious chronic illness called sarcoidosis was given.[2] This auto-immune disease was detected due to swollen lymph nodes in one of my lungs. Medical science has no known cause for the disease, hence no cure. Their only treatment is steroids. Ugh!

None of the three specialists who treated me during that time period—a cardiologist, pulmonary specialist and internal physician—ever suggested I change my diet to help rid the disease. However, I conducted my own research and began connecting the dots. I really didn't know what I was looking for; therefore, I didn't find much that could relieve my symptoms of occasional sharp chest pains and compromised breathing. At one point, the muscles in my legs were so weakened I had to be carried up/down the stairs, otherwise crawl. I had no relief except for my faith.

Speaking of which, here is where I put my faith in supernatural healing. I believe just as God gives us the power to get wealth, He gives us the power to be healed. However, that power requires more of us than just praying. For instance, should a person who prays all day for healing from cancer, all the while continuing to eat foods with ingredients known to fuel the growth of cancer cells, expect to become cancer free?

I suppose that person could expect their answered prayers to come in the form of radiation treatments and surgery. Yes, burning and carving of the body. Seems much harsher than simply eating nutritious meals for one's true healing—yet, *I'm* the crazy one.

The Universe already has everything in answer to our prayers before we even pray them. Therefore, our only prayer should be to have the *willpower* to seek out the answer and the *wisdom* to recognize it and receive it when it's dropped into our lap. That's when full manifestation of that which we are believing for can occur.

---

[1] *See Appendix A. Page 95. Figure 1.*
[2] *Ibid. Page 95.*

4

Based on my extensive nutritional research, it appears the answer regarding disease prevention and elimination is in Mother Nature—real food that the Earth springs forth. It's what I refer to as food before man puts his grubby hands in the mix and adds hormones, pesticides, chemicals, additives, toxins and other disease-causing elements for the sake of mass productivity, preservation and profit.

So, in the course of our praying for healing from diseases we must put the bad food aside. That's what I began doing after reading everything I could get my hands on about sarcoidosis in the early 2000's.

In 2003, while living in the Dallas-Fort Worth, Texas area, God led a beautiful couple from Mississippi into my presence, Bill and Joyce Frederick. Following their lead from their extensive research on candida yeast in the body, I stopped consuming white sugar, white flour, white potatoes, white rice and white bread. I nixed starches and hydrogenated fats as much as I knew how, which, in hindsight, wasn't much since they're well hidden in so many processed foods. That caused my symptoms to lessen at a faster rate than any of the 15 different medications those three doctors had prescribed for me!

However, over the next nine years, I still periodically dealt with shortness of breath when climbing stairs; swollen ankles (due to poor blood circulation) when sitting too long; and occasional severe chest pains that would stop me cold in my tracks. What excruciating pain! I now know that all those symptoms had everything to do with my bad habits of poor dietary choices, lack of sleep, inconsistent exercising and the allowance of the big "s," stress.

Fast forward to August 2012

In 2012, God once again brought someone across my path to shed tremendous light on my food intake in relation to my health issues: Keidi Awadu, aka Chef Keidi. He and I actually knew each other as small children 50 years prior but hadn't interacted since. In the late 1950's and early 60's, our mothers were best friends until the untimely death of his mother when he was age seven. That makes our recent match up truly made in heaven (but that story is for another book).

5

I had recently moved to the West Coast when he popped up on my radar, living only about 300 miles from me. Chef Keidi introduced me to his book, *Living Superfood Recipes*, and his raw, superfoods dietary lifestyle. That was the first time I recall hearing the term raw foodist. It soon became clear that as a raw foodist, or rawtarian—which is what I prefer to be called—I would be adopting a more scientific approach to eating than a vegan would.

I took a one-month crash course on "real food vs. fake food" using Chef Keidi's impressive 30+ years of researched information on nutrition being compiled for his book, *Living Superfood Research*, published in 2014. Currently, there are a total of four books in the Living Superfood Series: *Living Superfood Recipes, Living Superfood Research, Living Superfood Longevity* and *Living Superfood Recipes Volume 2*.

As a result of that research, I went from eating a modified Standard American Diet one day to eating raw, plant-based meals the very next day. Yes, it was that quick of a transition because I was sick and tired of being sick and tired. I drew a line in the sand and never looked back! I call it my SAD to RAW transformation.

Even with my food restrictions implemented in 2003, I had never been a vegan or vegetarian. In fact, I don't think I personally knew a vegan or vegetarian back then. After all, I lived in Texas. That is one meat-eating state! I believe meat ranks right up there with religion with most people in that Bible-Belt region. We mustn't forget what happened to Oprah when she made one simple statement denouncing a hamburger!

All I knew was that for my health's sake, it wasn't a matter of whether or not I *wanted* to change the way I ate; I *had* to change. Is change a hard thing to do? Of course, it is but here's how I approach almost every difficult task requiring major effort on my part. I ask myself these two questions and answer them as well: Was childbirth hard? You bet it was—both times! Was the outcome great? Most definitely—both times! I ended up a better person for it, as well. Case closed.

With that frame of mind, onward I marched with my transformation to a healthier me. I eliminated ALL foods that required cooking. That meant I ate nothing fried, baked, boiled, broiled, bbq'd, sauteed, nuked, steamed, poached, wok'ed, or otherwise. That also meant getting rid of my microwave.

In the past, if anyone had told me I'd be functioning without a microwave oven, I would have called them crazy. I even heated my water in the microwave. Yet, here I am in 2017, five years later still without one in the house and still vowing to never use one again. I've learned that microwave ovens offer more than just heating foods and what that "more" consists of "ain't good." Mainly, microwave cooking changes the nutrients in the food causing unhealthy changes in the user's blood. Over time, this could lead to the deterioration of the human system.

I purchased Chef Keidi's *Living Superfood Recipes* book right away, but can I be honest with you? I opened it and became overwhelmed. I didn't know how *I* could prepare any of those dishes. The pictures of his food looked great on his website and in the recipe book. To hear him tell it, it was fairly easy to make all those dishes.

However, anyone who knows me knows that the kitchen had never been my favorite room in the house. It was perhaps my least favorite. Generally, I'd go in there to toss something in the oven or microwave and then quickly leave to do something more important until the food was finished—or burnt, if I forgot to set a timer.

But I knew I had to persevere in this raw venture; I had to get results. Therefore, I had to make peace with the kitchen. I got in there and started juicing. That seemed simple enough since I had a blender. I did not have a food dehydrator nor a food processor, so a lot of those other dishes in the recipe book would have to wait. The important thing was that I started.

Too often people don't do *anything* because they're not sure how to do *everything*. I've been guilty of that a time or two in many facets of my life. But no more, where my health is concerned. I had to take action if I wanted to get well. I had to create a paradigm shift; a mind reset. Only then could my body follow.

My Light Bulb Moment

After a couple weeks of juicing and trying several simple recipes from his recipe book, I traveled to the city where Chef Keidi lived and had the pleasure of tasting a "feast" prepared especially for me. My plate had eight to ten

7

different items on it, not counting the several desserts that came afterward.

Everything tasted amazingly delicious! That was the moment I became instantly sold on raw, living super foods!

That was also the moment a light bulb came on in my head and I suddenly realized what was happening. I was giving my body the enzymes, proteins and nutrients it was designed to have all along in order to operate optimally and fight off diseases. Just the enzymes alone can make a huge difference in helping the body do what it is supposed to do: heal itself.

Within seven days of eating *full* plates of these live enzyme-rich meals, I noticed a significant change. ALL my sarcoidosis symptoms disappeared! That's right, in just seven days! But don't take my word for it, try it yourself and see.

I'm not talking about eating little veggie snacks, or the same old boring salad and veggie juices like I started off doing. No, I'm talking about turning your meals into orthomolecular medicine—delicious medicine at that. This process of healing all the way down to one's cellular level with nutrients, proteins, minerals and vitamins is no respecter of person. That means if it harvested a positive outcome for me it will do the same for you!

I decided to write the first version of this book (an e-book published in 2014) after completing one year of being a rawtarian and engaging in seasonal detoxification fasts. In addition to all sarcoidosis symptoms going away in those first seven days, throughout that first year, pesky menopausal nuances lessened tremendously and I "offed" 30 pounds (a few of which I since gained back but that's okay). That brought me down four dress sizes —effortlessly. So, why would I ever go back to my old way of eating?

Before and After

No matter how great our testimony is of adopting a healthier lifestyle, before-and-after photos tend to be the real proof. I happen to have a couple photos of me wearing the same pair of pants years apart. They have since become the measuring stick of my weight loss achievement upon going raw.[3]

[3] See Appendix B. Page 99

In the fall of 2007, I borrowed my daughter's pair of capris to wear on a cruise to the West Indies. They fit a little snug, as my daughter weighed less than me, but sufficed, nonetheless. Unfortunately, I don't have any photos of me wearing them on the cruise.

Eight months later, when warm weather finally arrived in the Midwest (where I lived at the time), I attempted to wear those same capris and was quite dismayed that I couldn't. I took a photo displaying how they fit—or should I say didn't fit—while also displaying a staged look of shock. My shameless eating binge on that cruise, having rich desserts with almost every meal, started my body on a course I couldn't easily reverse. I had added seven pounds in those eight months! No doubt, the bulk of it occurring right on that ship.

At 147 pounds, I felt sluggish and unlovely. I'm only 5'2", so that's a body mass index (BMI) of 26.9%, indicating a very overweight situation. I wasn't even that heavy when nine months pregnant with either child! Yep, this was my all-time heaviest weight.

What had really gotten me started on this weight-gaining path was steroids prescribed to me in 2000 for the sarcoidosis. Even though I refused to take them past a couple weeks of 40 milligrams per day dosage, the damage weight-wise (as well as other ways internally, I'm sure) was already done. In 2001, my weight had gotten to 140 pounds and stayed.

So, that photo showed me I needed to take action, and quick. Since I already knew what to do regarding cutting out meat, sugar, carbs and such, I once again tried to eat sensibly. What really is sensibly, though, when you don't know what you don't know? My efforts did help me drop about 10 pounds but I found it next to impossible to get any lower than my 137 to 140-pound range.

In 2011, when my daughter was in college, I came across those capris again packed away in her closet. I tried them on for the heck of it and was pleasantly surprised that I could at least fasten them. I wouldn't wear them in public, though, with such a muffin top going on! Sigh.

Three years later, I had completed my raw transformation and what came across my path? You guessed it, those same capris. By now, I'm sure they're not reappearing in my life by accident, so of course I had to try them on. This time, they fit quite fine on my redefined and fabulous body! Zipping up with ease and no muffin top. Now, we're talking! I vowed to keep these capris as my weight gauge every three years from now to forever!

Chapter 2
Raw Intelligence

When I started this raw food journey, I was just finishing my second master's degree program—this one in Health Law at Loyola University, Chicago School of Law. I was immersed in health care information: the administrative side of it; the legislative side of it; the financial side of it; the medical personnel side of it; the information technology side of it; and the ethics side of it. All those lectures I sat through and all that research I conducted opened my eyes wide. Hence, I felt there were three important personal decisions I needed to make. That is, if I considered myself an intelligent person—which I did and do.

My first decision dealt with hospitals: I needed to stay out of them at all cost!

In 2011, at the beginning of my second year of that master's program, I spent several days as a patient in ICU. I went to the ER with excruciating chest pains and difficulty breathing due to a sarcoidosis episode. While the medical staff watched my oxygen levels in ICU, I interviewed my nurses and received a firsthand account—albeit a small glimpse—of the state of our nation's hospital system.

The next day after I was released from the hospital, my best friend of 38 years died from pancreatic cancer following surgery in a hospital a thousand miles away. Her doctor later admitted he misdiagnosed her illness until it was too late to save her. I didn't get to see her in her final stage of life. Worse than that, I was her Medical Power of Attorney, yet I was not there prior to the surgery to help her make decisions or to act on her behalf. The very surgery from which she never recovered could've possibly been avoided.

I'm not sure if I've forgiven myself yet for not being there for her. If I had taken better care of myself by eating better, I would not have been confined. I cannot be useful to *anyone* when stuck in a hospital bed—not to my children, my friends, nor my family. After learning of her death, I vowed to never again be stuck in a hospital bed.

My second decision also dealt with hospitals: I needed to teach others to stay out of them!

I had just learned in my studies that according to a 2000 IOM (Institute of Medicine) Report, as many as 98,000 people die in any given year from *preventable* medical errors that occur in hospitals. That's more than the number of people who die from motor vehicle accidents, breast cancer, or AIDS—three causes that receive far more public attention! In 2008, The U.S. Department of Health and Human Services Office reported 180,000 deaths by medical error among Medicare patients alone. In a 2016 study by Johns Hopkins, it was estimated that a whopping 251,454 deaths are attributed to medical errors annually in the United States. So, there you have it. A major problem that is truly escalating not dissipating.

Two of my theses written towards my law degree dealt with hospitals. The first paper was entitled, *Our US Health Care System's New ICU: Intrinsic Castration of the Underserved*. My final thesis expounded on that theme. It was entitled, *Racial Disparities in US Health Care Demands Competency and Legislative Repair*.

People need to listen to what experts are saying about hospitals. By experts, I mean medical scientists, biochemists, biomedical engineers and researchers, clinical professors, certified nutritionists, naturopathic specialists, as well as progressively thinking physicians and other clinicians. So, when these experts say the cure is not in the meds but in the food we eat, why is there still disbelief among the people?

I read an article by a nurse of 22+ years who served in various countries and capacities. She's a best-selling author who has conducted numerous TV and radio interviews. She states that hospitals are lacking a fundamental component to ensure a better healthcare model: the use of nutritious living foods to supplement and enhance the healing of those within the hospital's care.[4]

If experts are saying nutrition belongs in the hospitals, why aren't patients holding their hospitals accountable, instead of allowing themselves to be fed the same damaging food that got them in there in the first place? I ask this question from an intelligence standpoint, all the while realizing people relate subconsciously to food from an emotional standpoint. The very food that people should be staying away from is inhibiting them from making the wise decision to do so.

I know it's quite a stretch for me to think a lack of nutrition in hospitals is enough to convince you and others to stay out of there. So, how about then letting those statistics of death by medical errors—otherwise known as iatrogenic—guide your decision? Let those statistics outrage you to the point of action. That action being staying healthy; hence, clear of hospitals.

My third decision dealt with my diet and exercise: I needed to improve them!

I had already been writing health newsletters/blogs since 2001. My first newsletter was called Three Step Healing. It focused on pairing up knowledge of supernatural healing with the practical steps needed to ensure wellness. Back then, I knew nothing about eating only a plant-based diet, but I wrote often about cutting certain things out of one's diet, like sugars, caffeine, additives, etc.

In July 2012, I suffered another sarcoidosis episode and didn't tell anyone about it. Over the past 12 years of dealing with that horrible chronic disease, that flare-up ranked rather high on the pain scale. Chest pains on and off, shortness of breath, swollen ankles; I had it all. I stuck to my vow of not

---

[4] Berkley, J. (2014, Vol. 33 Is. 4). When Hospitals Get it, I'll be Right There. *Healing Our World*, 30-31.

going to a hospital, though, and instead just prayed for relief. After a day or so, the pain subsided.

About a month later, I was introduced to the idea of eating raw, plant-based foods with live enzymes. Talk about an answered prayer! (For a full account of how it all transpired see Chapter 1, *MY TESTIMONY*.)

So, RAW it was for me. I had learned the science behind the molecular structural damage that occurs to the cells in our body due to the heating process of foods. I had learned how plant-based food consumption fights disease from an orthomolecular level. I had learned that the toxic additives of GE (genetically engineered) food and GMOs (genetically modified organisms), whereby genes from one organism are introduced into the DNA of another organism to resist pathogens and herbicides, are causing death and disease to our global population at an alarming rate.

Most importantly, I learned to make intelligent—not emotional—choices about eating. In doing so, I'm not denying myself anything, but granting myself ALL the benefits that a rejuvenated body has to offer.

I got sick and tired of being sick and tired, so I drew a line in the sand! I chose RAW: to **R**each **A**nd **W**in. I know you can do the same to achieve *your* disease-free and rejuvenated body!

> "We have lost an entire generation health-wise… with 35 diseases tied to GE crops."
>
> —Dr. Don Huber, Purdue University

> "Sufficient research on GE foods has been completed enough to conclude that GE foods are an explicit danger to human health, the living ecology of the planet and the literal survival of the species. Approximately 62 nations have already banned or mandated labeling of GE foods—wake up, America—let's take action!"
>
> —Gabriel Cousens, MD

Chapter 3
Going Raw

So what does it mean to "go raw" and why would you even want to?

First of all, I've learned not to broadcast the fact I eat raw. First of all, for most people I've encountered, that term has never registered on their radar. If they have heard it, they never ventured into learning what it entails. Secondly, for those who do know about it, the moment they learn I'm a rawtarian, they immediately think I'm going to judge what they're eating. They will say things like, *"Don't look at my plate!"* or *"I tried that once and it was great, but my body craves meat."*

In my mind I say, *"Oh boy, here we go again."*

So, unless I'm presenting at a health-related event or on video and the topic is food, I don't like to just come into the room as "the rawtarian." Surprisingly, though, that is how others see me and how some introduce me. When I'm meeting someone through a mutual friend, that friend may say, *"This is Terri. She's a rawtarian."* Or, *"This is Terri. She eats only raw foods."*

At this point in my raw journey (five years), I don't mind that type of introduction. I'm perhaps even amused or flattered by it. However, I just don't want people thinking that because of this healthier lifestyle I've chosen I'm better than them or I'm judging them. I've just simply kicked the food addiction that they can kick as well—when they're ready.

Generally, though, once the introduction has been made that I'm eating raw, people will right away say, *"Oh, so you're vegan?"* Again, a big indication they don't have a clue what raw is.

"No, I'm not a vegan, I'm raw, as in uncooked, unprocessed, live enzymes and superfoods. It's a couple levels up from vegan." As I'm saying that, the person is slowly nodding their head with their eyes glazed over. They're either intrigued or they think I'm in some sort of eating cult. Mainly, they think I'm a weirdo meat protestor who's going to tell them why they're going to hell for killing innocent animals and eating their flesh. I want to assure them that that's more of what a vegan does, not me.

While I'm making light of it, I do know there is a seriousness to veganism. However, more and more, I realize that out there in this big world lies a misguided view of a vegan lifestyle. Shapeless clothing, ugly sandals, bland meals and questionable hygiene. That's the traditional image that may first pop into one's mind. Oh yeah, and they throw blood on people's fur coats.

Unfortunately, those are the images society paints. Other than that, I had no clue about vegans because I never paid attention to their lifestyle. You see, when I came into raw eating, I had never been a vegetarian or a vegan. I went raw "cold turkey" style (pun intended). Prior to that, I had only modified my SADness (Standard American Diet) by cutting out most red meats, a lot of sugar and starches and by eating at a vegetarian restaurant from time to time while living in Chicago.

Modified SAD meant I still enjoyed my glass of Pepsi very often. It meant I still lusted after Chicago deep dish pizza and Breyers' vanilla bean ice cream. It meant I savored every bite of my mom's most-delicious-on-this-earth cobblers. Yum, yum! Some modification, huh?

Now that I am raw, I've learned a thing or two about vegans. I know they make conscious choices regarding their diets, yet a large percentage of them still get sick. Some even acquire the same death-threatening illnesses that meat-eaters are prone to. Why? Because their tired and overworked liver and pancreas are still having to deal with the cooked pasta and bread intake, which is boosting the sugar level, boosting the insulin and gluing up the insides with gluten.

So, I have a hard time understanding going through all those measures to cut out *some* things from my diet and still not gain a healthier advantage over carnivores. If I'm going to make changes to get healthy, I'm going to make sure the changes I make are actually going to do the job all the way.

Truth is, everyone has varying degrees of commitment. I'm not to judge whether someone else's commitment is right for them or the best they can do. However, when I said there's a seriousness—or conscientiousness, if you will—to veganism, it seems to me that it lies more in their ethical reasons than their health reasons.

I applaud vegans and their ethical choices in all aspects of their life. They typically have a strong conviction to not eat anything that "has a mother" or "that has eyes." Mainly, they don't want to contribute to the exploitation of animals, since they are innocent beings. Hey, I can get behind all that. Makes complete sense.

However, I cannot get behind the notion that eating as a vegan, or pescatarian (the newest addition to the food hierarchy, as one who eats like a vegan but adds fish to their diet), is going to prevent diseases and illnesses. It just doesn't line up with the nutritional research that's out there. But, to each his own, right? As long as one is *not* looking to prevent disease and illness, then carry on with veganism! There's great value to it, nonetheless.

For me, going raw means I have eliminated from my regular diet approximately 98% of foods that are cooked or processed. That means I avoid the pastas, breads, potatoes and other dangerous starches that even vegans still eat. In essence, 98% of the time I don't eat anything fried, baked, boiled, broiled, bbq'd, sauteed, nuked, steamed, poached or wok'ed. In that 2%, where I will eat something cooked or processed due to a particular situation, those food items will more than likely never be fried and never consist of meat. That's just too big of a risk for me to take.

Going raw means I choose to eat foods full of LIVE enzymes, proteins, minerals and nutrients so that my body operates at its optimum capacity.

It has more to do with the science behind how my body prevents diseases and heals itself, than how I am morally saving poor innocent pigs, chickens and chinchillas.

Going raw means, I have become fully and consciously aware of what I'm putting into this God-given temple of mine. Eating intelligently, instead of from an emotional standpoint, is also a far less selfish way of existing for many proven reasons.

So why would *you* want to go raw? I don't know; why would you?

Ethical reasons?

• Millions of animals are being tortured in factory farms and slaughterhouses. They are kept in tiny, filthy cages, unable to move for the majority of their lives. They are beaten, drugged and abused. Our government offers weak regulations at best, allowing these horrible conditions to become acceptable.

• Slaughterhouses' working conditions are super dangerous. Workers are exposed to sharp items, high temperatures, and bodily fluids of animals that could potentially carry disease. Employees are typically ex-convicts, illegal residents and the like who cannot defend their own rights. As long as high demand for meat products continues, those conditions will most likely continue as well.

Environmental reasons?

• Almost half of the fossil fuels produced in the US are used to raise animals for food.

• Inadequate sewer systems throughout our country allow animal waste to "run-off" into nearby bodies of water and food crops. This excrement is more concentrated than human feces and is often contaminated with herbicides, pesticides, hormones, antibiotics, etc.

Health reasons?

• Meat eaters are prone to obesity nine times more than non-meat eaters. Science has shown that obesity is a basis for mineral deficiency. Almost all illnesses and diseases leading to premature death can be traced to mineral deficiency.

• The consumption of meat, eggs, wheat, dairy products and the artificial additives and preservatives used in processed foods has also been strongly linked to diabetes, heart disease, osteoporosis, various cancers, Alzheimer's, asthma, and infertility.

• Many people have successfully reversed and prevented disease and chronic illness through a full spectrum of minerals, proteins and highly nutrient-dense super foods diet.

• Eating solely based on emotion—what I call reckless eating—allows illnesses traditionally known as geriatric diseases to now come upon people in their 50's, 40's and sometimes even younger. Just think about the astronomical cost of medical treatment required to keep people alive for the last 30+ years of their lives! Money that is being handed over to the medical industry, instead of into the coffers of people's heirs. Doesn't the Bible say that a good man leaves an inheritance for his children and his children's children? Oh, but that's right, God must not have known anything about the evils of cancer and heart disease when He laid down that command.

Chapter 4
It's Not Only About Nutrition

While what we're shoveling down our pie hole has a lot to do with how we're feeling and how our body is functioning, it's only one piece of the puzzle of wellness. There are several other important factors that I would be remiss if I didn't mention. In addition to good nutrition, they are proper hydration, adequate sleep, emotional well-being, strong spiritual orientation, regular exercise and stress management. These factors all work hand-in-hand to keep you fit and fabulous.

They are listed here in no particular order of importance. In one brief statement, here's how, in my opinion, each will benefit you:

- Good nutrition – Our body uses food for energy and for healing itself. If you're eating a standard American diet (SAD), anywhere from 40-80% of your body's energy goes towards digesting. When we give our body the enzymes, proteins and nutrients it needs to operate optimally, that digestion process is sped up, reserving the body's energy to fight off diseases.

- Proper hydration – Our body consists of over 70% water. Every cell in our body needs oxygen to function properly. That oxygen (O) is delivered to those cells by way of water, (H_2O). No oxygen? Then you have abnormal cell function. Abnormal cells are cancerous cells. Cancerous cells form clusters called tumors.

- Adequate sleep – During sleep, our body repairs itself. Lack of sleep, lack of repairing. Over time, lack of repairing leads to a weakened immune system that is incapable of fighting off infection and disease. Going to bed and rising at the same time each day, maintaining our circadian rhythm, helps to fight diseases like obesity, diabetes, depression, bipolar disorder and seasonal affective disorder.

- Emotional well-being – Being sad and angry zaps a whole lot of energy from our body. Again, just as with digesting good nutritious food, when you're happy instead of sad or angry, you are freeing up energy that the body can now use for more important things like keeping our organs operating at their optimum level.

- Spiritual orientation – Having a strong spiritual life goes a long way in helping us overcome life's adversities. It brings us hope for a brighter tomorrow, allows us to have faith in a source much larger than ourselves and teaches us the power of unconditional love.

- Regular exercise – Medical studies have proven that sitting is the new cigarette smoking. Our physical inactivity presents a major risk for heart disease. To turn that around, exercising a minimum of 20 to 30 minutes per day at least three times a week decreases that risk drastically.

- Stress management – Stress is a silent killer. When our body goes into high stress, our cortisol levels are raised (called fight or flight). When this hormone remains raised for long periods of time, it wreaks havoc on our entire immune system.

Let's take a look at just one piece of the healthy lifestyle puzzle: stress. I've found that a very effective way to combat stress is through writing therapy. As an avid journaler of many years, writing my feelings down may come more natural to me than to someone who has never kept a diary or journal, or worse yet, to someone who is tied to their technology and thinks that writing is old fashioned. They may be very surprised to learn medical studies have proven that anyone suffering from stress, depression or a myriad of health challenges can benefit from writing—not typing—their thoughts on paper.

Journaling can be the breeding ground for positive ideas and thoughts to flush out old, negative ones. It can bring about strength for a newly-inspired lifestyle

I am humbled by one of the survey responses to a journaling workshop I conducted years ago. It stated, *"Terri's style of presentation makes journaling a less tedious process and an activity [that] can be used by all people for self-reflection and healing."* Self-reflection, which leads to self-healing really is the main therapeutic usefulness of journaling.

In my opinion, we can never do enough self-reflection or introspection, which is the detailed mental examination of our feelings, thoughts and motives. Take, for instance, the question, *"How are you?"* Three simple words. We perhaps speak them multiple times per day; basically, each time we greet someone. Imagine, now, the inner reflection that would take place if we were to ask ourselves that same question AND answer it. Generally, we're too busy to ask that of ourselves, let alone answer it.

I challenge you to reach deep inside for a little emotional detoxification through journaling. Discovering how you are really doing inside empowers you to embrace these three options to go from victim to victor in any situation: 1) change it, 2) accept it, or 3) leave it.

Part II

My Transformation

Chapter 5
Gaining Knowledge

When I first went raw, I had no idea how much I didn't know about food —real food, that is. I soon found out there was plenty to learn. I'm still learning today, five years later. I'll still be learning for years to come. I love that about this lifestyle. It's always pushing me to go deeper and higher for my health's sake.

Sifting through mounds of notebooks and computer files kept since starting this journey to decide what important information to include in this book proved a daunting task, as everything is important! If I included it all, I'd be writing forever. So, I picked several topics that seem to come up a lot in conversations I have with individuals attempting to adopt a healthier lifestyle.

Hopefully, these are things you had questions about as well and will now have a slightly better understanding. At the very least, perhaps it will prompt you to look further into these and other healthy matters.

Enzymes

As I mentioned earlier, as soon as I began eating full, nutrient-dense, plant-based superfood-rich meals, I felt amazing! I was instantly sold on raw, living Superfoods. I described it as a light bulb coming on in my head as I suddenly realized what was happening inside every organ of my body. I was giving my body all the proteins, minerals, and other nutrients that it was designed to have in order to operate optimally and fight off diseases.

27

I began to look into this intriguing world of one particular protein, enzymes. The spelling of the name alone, with its "z" and "y" in the middle, seemed fascinating enough to me. I discovered there are thousands of chemical reactions taking place in our body every second to keep it functioning properly. One such function, as a result of chemical reactions, is where the body turns food into energy.

The raw foods I am now consuming on a regular basis contain live enzymes that help speed up this process. Without enzymes in the food to speed up these chemical reactions, the digestive enzymes are left to break down food at a much slower pace. This causes a burden on the whole digestive system and the intestines, as they are then required to work overtime in an attempt to turn that food into energy.

If you're ever wondering why you're feeling tired and sluggish day in and day out, it's time to take a long hard look at what you're eating. Chances are you're giving your intestines, liver, pancreas, gallbladder and even your rectum a workout they weren't equipped for.

Proteins

One of the most frequently asked questions I have received on this raw journey of mine by far has been: *"If you don't eat meat, where are you going to get your proteins from?"* I have had people passionately debate me regarding their "you need meat for protein" stance. Even as a newbie Superfoods researcher my argument held up against theirs strictly on logic.

So, this one piece of logic halts all arguments. I answer their question with these series of questions: "Where does the cow get its protein from? Where does the gorilla get its protein from? Where does one of the strongest animals in the kingdom, the elephant, get its protein from?" These are all big and strong herbivores who survive and thrive without eating dead flesh. Undeniably, they get their proteins from plants, as I now do.

All plants are comprised of proteins, some in a more concentrated manner than others. Some plants are so dense with proteins that they contain fiber, vitamins, omega fats and essential micronutrients not ever found in meat. Sea vegetation, like spirulina and chlorella, is one such powerful source. This species has the highest concentration of proteins among all plants.

According to the book, *The Blue Zones*, there are specific places in the world that experience the highest percentage of people living astoundingly longer than anyone else. They are not feeble either, but full of vitality well into their 80's, 90's and 100s. One such group of people is from Okinawa, Japan about 1000 miles from Tokyo. As the longest living people, they also have the greatest number of disease-free and disability-free people comparing with all men at an average age of 72.3 and with all women at an average age of 77.7. Their centenarian ratio, the highest in the world, is five per every 10,000 people.[5]

What does the Okinawa's diet consist of? Mainly, sea vegetation, their favorite dish being a spam and vegetable stir-fry. Traditionally, the elders have never had coca cola, hamburgers, junk food or rich foods. Instead, they ate from their gardens filling up on things like daikon, bitter melon, garlic, onion, peppers, and tomatoes to complement their fish and tofu. A country-wide favorite for all three meals per day prior to WWII was imo, a type of sweet potato. They are super high in vitamin C and fiber, as well as beta-carotene.[6]

As great as their diet is, there is more to their longevity than just a high concentration of proteins through plants. Remember I mentioned in Chapter 4 that healthy is more than just nutrition—it's a complete lifestyle. A typical day for the Okinawan includes a nap, tinkering in the garden, time spent with loved ones and bedtime by 9pm.[7]

Amino acids

Back to the question of, *"Where are you going to get your proteins from?"* When someone asks this question, they've perhaps heard a meat advocate argument the point about meat containing protein and decided that must be the gospel truth. But if you were to ask them what a protein is, you would quickly see they don't have a leg to stand on regarding their meat argument.

---

[5] Buettner, Dan, (2008). *The Blue Zones*. National Geographic. Page 68.

[6] Ibid. Page 84.

[7] Ibid. Page 84.

Here's what a protein is (since you probably won't learn it from that person arguing their meat case): Proteins are amino acids that are joined together to form a chain. Some proteins are just a few amino acids long; others are made up of thousands of amino acids. Now, you may be asking what is an amino acid? This amino acid building block is a simple organic compound that forms together to give our cells their structure. They are essential for every metabolic process that takes place in our body.

Therefore, the correct question someone should ask you when they are puzzled about you eating a raw diet is, *"Where are you going to get your 20 essential amino acids from?"* Most are produced right inside your body. However, out of the 20, there are eight or nine amino acids that we must get from outside the body. These are found abundantly in plants—soybeans as well as veggies.

Antioxidants

Antioxidants are substances that are anti (against) oxidants (oxidation). So, they are crucial in the healing process as it relates to repairing cell damage caused by oxidation in the body. This oxidative state occurs when certain types of oxygen molecules are allowed to float freely in the body forming free radicals.

What are free radicals? They are atoms or groups of atoms containing unpaired electrons. They are formed when oxygen interacts with certain molecules, causing a highly reactive chain reaction. A great example of this is what happens with iron over time when exposed to water.

Antioxidants go throughout your body like little scavengers attacking free radicals to help prevent cell damage and reverse any damage already done. There are endogenous antioxidants that are created inside our body and exogenous antioxidants created outside our body. The most exogenous substances that contain antioxidant attributes are vitamins A, C and E as well as beta-carotene and lycopene.

Vitamin C is the most abundant water-soluble antioxidant. Vitamin E is the most abundant fat-soluble antioxidant you can have in your body. Now, you are probably asking what is water soluble and fat soluble and how does each function? Well, you are very smart to ask that question.

30

Water soluble vitamins, such as B complex vitamins and vitamin C, dissolve in water. If you have excess amounts in your body, they are excreted through the kidneys. Fat-soluble vitamins–primarily vitamins A, D, E and K–dissolve in fat and are stored in fat throughout the body. The thing to watch out for with fat soluble vitamins is that they are difficult for your body to excrete. So, if you have them in excess from consuming too much, toxic levels can accumulate.

A sampling of foods and herbs rich in antioxidants:

Top 10 foods highest in antioxidants

1. Goji berries
2. Blueberries
3. Blackberries
4. Dark chocolate
5. Pecans
6. Artichoke
7. Elderberries
8. Kidney beans
9. Cranberries
10. Cilantro

Top 10 herbs highest in antioxidants

1. Clove
2. Cinnamon
3. Oregano
4. Turmeric
5. Cocoa
6. Cumin
7. Parsley (dried)
8. Basil
9. Ginger
10. Thyme

Herbivores vs. carnivores

It has been scientifically proven that humans are herbivores, plant eaters. Period. Therefore, we are herbivores, who, over time, evolved into enjoying a carnivore lifestyle. Did this lifestyle come out of necessity? I'm not an expert on any such theory to answer that; however, I just showed you how a plant-based diet provides all the adequate proteins for a 400-pound gorilla to thrive for many years.

If meat is not necessary in our diet to survive, why do so many people swear by it? My guess is habit and emotion. If someone was thinking outside of emotion, as in thinking logically, they would consider that the dangers of toxins and parasites in meat far outweigh any nutritional value given to it. You don't think there are any dangers in meat? Try eating yours uncooked.

Bottom line, our bodies were not created as a meat-eating species. Any Christian can follow their Bible, their sacred guide for living, to determine that—starting with Genesis 1:29. God makes it quite clear the role that plants, NOT meat, has in our lives for sustainability purposes. As Chef Keidi often quips, *"There was no convection oven tree in the Garden of Eden, nor was there a microwave bush."*

How we got to this place of acting like carnivores seems quite complicated. Nevertheless, we're here and it's wrecking lives like crazy. First, the very notion of expecting our digestive system to handle the breaking down of dead carcass the same way a lion, wolf, vulture, or other true carnivore would break it down is ludicrous. Secondly, because our digestive system is *not* designed the same way as a carnivore's digestive system, a person who does choose to eat meat is simply aging their body at a faster rate than a person who doesn't. With this aging comes sickness, disease, and early death.

Let's put the meat vs. plant argument to rest with this simple comparison. Greens match every essential element the human body needs to live in optimum health. Everything, that is, except B-12. You will have to get that by supplementing your diet with vitamins.

On the other hand, here is what various meat components provide. Does meat provide protein? Yes. Does meat provide fiber? Nope. Does meat provide antioxidants, like vitamin C and vitamin B-12? Nope. Does meat provide Phyto-nutrients? Nope. Does meat provide live enzymes? Nope. Does meat provide oxygen? Nope.

Hmm. I think you'd better eat your greens!

Healing foods

Let's get it straight. Even though I wrote "healing foods," our bodies do all the healing—they were designed like that by our Creator. The food we put into our bodies either aid in that healing process, or they aid in the dying process. Here is a list of foods most commonly used in the healing process. This list is not by a long stretch an exhaustive list; however, there's plenty here for you to consume to get heading in the right direction.[8]

- Almonds
- Apples
- Asparagus
- Bananas
- Barley
- Celery
- Chocolate (cacao beans)
- Cinnamon
- Coconut
- Blackberries
- Blueberries
- Cabbage
- Carrots
- Cayenne
- Lettuce
- Oats
- Olives
- Oranges

---

[8] Awadu, Keidi. (2014) *Living Superfood Research*. Conscious Rasta Report. 149.

- Cranberries
- Dark leafy greens
- Dates
- Figs
- Garlic
- Ginger
- Grapes
- Green tea
- Lavender
- Legumes
- Lemons
- Parsley
- Pears
- Pineapple
- Prunes
- Rice
- Sage
- Sea vegetables
- Spinach
- Strawberries
- Turmeric
- Walnuts

My Journal Entries Regarding The Nutritional Knowledge I Gained

August 8, 2012

During several email exchanges and phone conversations, as Keidi and I became re-acquainted for the first time in 50 years, the subject of my health came up. After sharing with him about the heart attack I suffered at age 40, and the diagnosis of sarcoidosis (autoimmune disorder) I was given following that event, Chef Keidi, as he's known to the community due to his award-winning status as a raw food chef, sent me this email…

"I want to share some of what I think will help you immensely to overcome the immune challenge.

- As soon as possible, you should transition towards a whole food, live food lifestyle. It would not only be for your health's sake but for the future generations of your family.
- Green juicing is the fastest course to the greatest degree of release. You would also be best to incorporate a seasonal detoxification program which will do a number of things positively to your whole body systems to bring them into balance and optimized function.

- It is generally recommended that people increase their vitamin D intake to boost the immune system. In the case of autoimmune diseases this is NOT the case as a boost in the immune system is not moving in the direction towards balance that is needed. Because of this, many times people with lupus, sarcoidosis or other autoimmune disorders are best to avoid excess direct sunshine, which generates vitamin D.

- There is a common problem in sarcoidosis patients with the exchange of oxygen and carbon dioxide resulting in the depth of breathing being severely restricted. I've recently come across the work of Konstantin Buteyko, a Russian scientist who had developed a revolutionary breathing technique which was said to create healing miracles. (You can learn more about these techniques on YouTube under Buteyko.)"

I appreciated his helpful information and resources and chose not to be offended by his unsolicited advice. After all, an offended spirit cannot learn or receive anything. Since I had been praying for relief from that illness, I needed to receive the answer to that prayer any way God chose to bring it. Nutritional change was God's answer, which is why two weeks later, I went ALL RAW and got ALL HEALED.

May 15, 2013

It's grocery shopping day. My grocery bills have been slashed in half since going raw. Cutting out processed foods works wonders for the budget!

Unfortunately, people have been brainwashed to believe it is too expensive to eat healthy. On the contrary! First, we know the terribly high, crippling cost of being sick in America. Secondly, we know (or should know) bad food leads to being obese and eventually sick. Therefore, an easy math equation can help you figure out the rest. For example:

If $A = B$ and $B = C$, then $A = C$. If buying and eating healthy foods equals wellness and wellness equals huge savings from hospital bills and prescriptions; then buying and eating healthy foods equals savings.

There are ways to master grocery shopping for fruits and veggies to bring you even greater savings.

1) Plan ahead and shop during sale days by checking the circulars of two or three stores.

2) Purchase only fruits and veggies in season—they cost less.

3) Make friends with the produce manager at your favorite store. Stores are constantly switching out the produce off the shelves and bins. The very ripe items must be taken down and replaced with the newer stuff. Chances are they are going to toss that fruit out, so ask them to cut you a deal for it. That so-called rejected fruit is great for juicing!

4) Search for a Mexican grocery store in your area. Their fruit and veggies are usually cheaper every day—not just on sale days. They offer the same quality, if not better, than the large chains.

I come home on market day with bags and bushels of fruit and the total bill is usually under $20. That's right, seven to eight bags for under twenty dollars!

June 13, 2013

You wouldn't eat pig poop on purpose, would you?

Some people have told me they wouldn't dare eat a vegan or raw meal because they want their food to taste like "real" food.

That's such a funny statement because first of all, it's not their so-called "real" food that tastes good, it's the seasonings. Hello! Think I'm lying? Bake a chicken without a stitch of seasoning and see how much you enjoy eating it. Therefore, the same method of seasoning used to make the toxic dead carcass taste scrumptious makes the live plant-based meal just as lip-smacking good!

Secondly, if you think you're eating anything nutritious and "real" then you really need to do your homework! You are eating fake, manufactured substances.

Foods are being designed to tolerate high levels of pesticides; to last longer in the transport and shelving process; and to grow bigger faster. To accomplish all this, foods are being genetically modified. You have been hearing more of that buzz word, GMO, right? Well, all the fuss is about companies, such as Epicyte, a California based manufacturer who admitted inserting anti-sperm antibodies from human females in YOUR foods for growth purposes. Corn, with this spermicide developed in it, causes the semen in men to become sterile.

If that doesn't ruffle your feathers, or if that doesn't apply to you, then what do you think about a little pig feces in your fish? Feces is being fed to tilapia to make them grow bigger. Yuck! The FDA allows it! If that is not what you ordered on the menu, then you'd better start doing your research and stop being fooled into believing what you're eating is safe. Government agencies sure as heck do not care.

We have an amazingly miraculous body with trillions of intricate workings. This earthly temple God put us in control of deserves only the best. Don't you agree?

Chapter 6
Acting on What I Learned

Too often, when giving healthy tips (and I'm very careful these days to only share these tips when asked) I hear people say, *"Yeah, I know…"* Okay, they know, but they're still not advancing in their health. They're still performing the same old habits. And we have all heard the definition of insanity, right?

So, there comes a time when we must take action—yes, even if we don't know everything there is to know. Usually, we do know enough that it should get us questioning and seeking for more answers.

For instance, we know our economy is in bad shape deficit-wise. Shall we keep complaining about it with no substance behind our complaint? Or do we conduct a little research and find out what the numbers represent so we will know what we're really complaining about? According to *Living Superfood Research*, 17% of GDP, approximately $10,000 per person, is added to our economy's deficit due to diseases and premature deaths.[9] That represents a whole lot of BBQ, cookies, and diet soda!

Com'on folks, we must stop the madness! We must eat to live and shun food that is literally "to die for." Keeping that mantra of "eat to live" fresh in my mind helped me to take the bull by the horn and claim my health. Even with many opportunities to fall back to my old eating habits, continuing forward just made more sense.

In other words, I will no longer commit "Chewicide." I like that word Chef Keidi coined for his documentary's title. Its concept clearly depicts food as

---

[9] Awadu, Keidi (2014). *Living Superfood Research*. Conscious Rasta Press, 143.

the silent killer looming over our nation. While causing more and more people to become reliant upon our nation's health care system, this system is failing the American people miserably.

In August 2012, I traveled from Las Vegas, where I had been living for about a year, back to Chicago to defend my thesis at Loyola University, Chicago School of Law. That was the last step in receiving my second master's degree—this one in Health Law. As I rehearsed my information on disparities in the health care system, I was reminded of just how broken our health care system is. It is broken because mindsets about food are broken.

If people didn't need their chocolate, French fries, sodas, sugar fixes, and other junk, then they wouldn't need all that medicine they're taking. Period. If the powers-that-be within this system weren't so motivated by greed then our healthcare system would work for the benefit of most, if not all, patients.

Good doctors would not be losing their practices—causing a dangerous void in the system—if they were not caught under the debacle of ridiculously high insurance rates. Those rates would not be so high if there weren't so many malpractice suits because of botched liposuction procedures or gastric by-pass surgeries. Those types of surgical fixes are presented as "the answer" to obesity by the medical industry more times than nutrition ever is.

We all must take responsibility for our actions. For instance, it was ridiculous when that woman sued McDonald's (and won) because their hot coffee scorched her lap when she spilled it there. By the same token, neither should we blame McDonald's because their cheeseburgers made us gain weight.

McDonald's isn't the only one getting blamed. Too many people are dying too young and folks are blaming it on God. Yep, God did it. *"God plucked so-and-so from the earth for His heavenly garden."* What the heck? That is the craziest rationale for poor nutrition I have ever heard—and I do hear it often!

So, we want people to belong to a god who *makes* them suffer with excruciating pain and anguish; and who causes body parts to have to be cut open? Will we expect them to endure this for many years until this god finally decides to pluck them up from here? Most would say, *"No thank you,"* to that ideology. If Christians who speak this way paused for one minute to reflect on their words, I believe many eulogies would be rephrased.

Aside from birth defects and other unexplained maladies caused by mutated genes, chromosomes or whatever, how about we just accept the responsibility for early death? How about, knowingly (as with cigarette smoking) or unknowingly (as with food consumption) we caused our own diseases to occur and God just allowed it to happen? He has no choice but to allow it when the options we choose go against the blessings He intended for us.

Bottom line, heart disease, diabetes, high blood pressure, cancer, and loads of chronic disorders ARE preventable. They are also food related. Look up the research—it's all there for us to discover. So, let us stop blaming God at every funeral and instead, work on ending chewicide!

My Journal Entries Regarding How I Took Action

August 10, 2012

Elation! Finally finished the thesis I've been working on practically nonstop for months. (This was my final work to confirm my master's degree in Health Law from Loyola University Law School-Chicago, in Chicago, Illinois.)

Two years of learning so much about our health care industry from many angles: financial, legal, legislative, disparities, ethics, technology, administrative, and even the human suffering associated with it. Having learned what I've learned, having watched the documentaries I've watched, having attended the forums where I heard fellow students defend their thesis, I am convinced everyone should consider improving their eating habits! All 39 root diseases in the world can be traced to foods.

My goal is to help people stay out of hospitals at all cost! It was such an eye-opener, learning about the 200,000 deaths per year that occur to patients while in the hospital due to PREVENTABLE errors, oversights, and accidents. One lady, the subject in a documentary produced by Professor Timothy McDonald, believed if her 15-year-old son had been anywhere else besides in a hospital, he would still be alive today. Terribly heartbreaking! Not a dry eye in the room. I have lost loved ones that way, too.

Terri Eileen Liggins

My Health Care Business and Finance professor liked a term paper I wrote on a similar topic and offered me the opportunity to be published in the financial law journal he publishes. He wants me to expound on the topic and present it back to him. What an honor!

I wrote that paper from my heart because the numbers are stacked against people of color in under-served communities. It is so important they open their eyes and learn that hospitals are not their ticket to health. Emergency room doctors should not be used as preventive care physicians. Yet there is such a tremendous wall of rejection to such change.

I will keep fighting until patients learn they must become partners with their doctors; do their own research; and help their doctor help them. They cannot sit back and let doctors experiment on them just because s/he dons the white coat. The answer to health, vitality and longevity is not in the meds!

August 23, 2012

I enjoyed a fun girls' night out in Chicago! We went to Fogo De Chao, a popular restaurant chain known for its decadent meats. I don't know how in the world I got suckered into a steakhouse. But it was cool.

I enjoyed this restaurant's food 14 or so years ago in Dallas. This time, though, I didn't touch any of their many different choices of savory, fire-roasted meats that were served and sliced right at our table by those gaucho chefs (the Brazilian term for them). I gorged instead at their salad bar— from quite an extensive selection. Besides the processed cold cuts, there was plenty there to satisfy my taste buds. I must say, the delicious raw asparagus and I bonded very well that evening.

I am proud of myself that I made it through the meal without backsliding in my eating. Had a wonderful time! After all, it's about the good company you're with, right? Not just about what you are shoving into your pie hole.

August 25, 2012

I attended a wonderful graduation feast put on by the faculty and administrative staff of the Beasley Institute—Loyola's law school. A wonderful expensive-looking dinner catered to us in a chic place in Chicago's upscale Rush Street area. I could tell they spent a lot of money on those meals, yet there was only one thing I could eat—the salad.

Yasmine, an online classmate of mine, who sat next to me at our table, had studied for this degree from her home in Egypt. She and her family made the trip overseas for the graduation festivities. She wore a hijab, so I knew she was Muslim. I figured she and her husband, who joined her for dinner, weren't going to be able to eat everything on that plate since the meat for sure wasn't Halal (permissible by their laws). As it turned out, neither of them touched *anything* on their plates, except the salad.

For dessert, came this huge slice of decadent chocolate cake. O-M-G! It looked *soo* delicious but is *soo* damaging to your body's organs in *soo* many ways! Once again, the three of us passed on it. No fruit was offered as an alternative dessert item to that cake. Tsk, tsk.

I felt bad seeing so much expensive food going to waste. Oh well, I suppose Loyola's event planners—as with most event planners in America—could have done a better job of not serving 100% Standard American Diet (SAD).

How about a healthy alternative like this raw desert? It contains a natural chocolate crust topped with wonderful fresh fruit and a delicious homemade gluten-free, dairy-free sauce. Your taste buds win AND your body wins—all the way down to the cellular level!

August 31, 2012

I'm doing it! I'm doing it! My third day of juicing only—no food. Yea! So proud of myself! I juiced some concoction of blue berries, mangos and other stuff. I forget what. I call it my BERRY MANGALOW, as in Barry Manilow (I confess; I used to own some of his albums back in the 80's). Much like Manilow, this drink is eclectic with a sweet melody of flavors for the palate!

I'm determined to embrace this lifestyle. In doing so, I'm not denying myself anything, but granting myself ALL the benefits that a rejuvenated body can bring. Consuming raw, live, plant-based foods snuff out a vast number of diseases at the orthomolecular level. I dare someone to show me otherwise. At times, when I want something quick but don't feel like preparing a healthy meal, I can throw things into the blender. Juicing or making smoothies is also a fun and tasty way for children to get a glassful of veggies and fruits without knowing it. How cool is that?

September 9, 2012

Today, I ran up a flight of stairs with a heavy bag of camera equipment. Afterward, I did not have to stand still for several minutes to catch my breath as would normally be the case. In fact, in the past I would not have made it the whole way up while running!

That may not seem like much to most people but previously, due to sarcoidosis in my lung, I could not even WALK up a flight of stairs without being winded. Wow, the only difference has been my raw food regimen!

I have always believed that some of the foods we eat are killing us, now I'm my own witness to the fact that there are foods to eat that will HEAL us! I don't remember how many steps I ran up, but they led to a pedestrian bridge high across Las Vegas Blvd on The Strip, so we're not talking about a few steps here.

This is my first time making couscous tabouli—it's uncooked, remember. Wow, where's the Easy Button? This stuff is so good, too!

September 14, 2012

Studies as of 2009 showed that 145 million people in the U.S. (that is nearly half our population) were living with a chronic condition such as diabetes, heart disease, depression or asthma. This should be unacceptable by us!

Even sadder is that all four of those listed diseases ARE REVERSIBLE without medicine but most people don't believe it. If they did, they would start today eating their way to health instead of to early death.

Personally, it seems to me that people like their illnesses. They cling to those ailments and medicines and speak about them as their badges of honor.

If you're feeling a little insulted now, then I'm probably talking about you. If you want to prove me wrong about those badges of honor, just simply open your mind to the possibility of feeling good and healthy—like you felt when you were a highly energized 21-year-old! Open your mind to the truth that chances are what's ailing you IS reversible with yummy foods and delicious juices and smoothies!

I've gotten the hang of juicing now, having made my very first super food, nutritionally dense smoothie. Preparing it was as easy as 1-2-3.

October 2, 2012

We must take steps—baby steps—by any means possible to turn this disease epidemic around in this country. Unfortunately, it's a little too late for some adults, whose minds will remain forever brainwashed into believing they're eating real food.

However, it is not too late for our children. They do not know the difference between healthy and not healthy. They simply desire something that tastes good and is perhaps fun like a Happy Meal™. So, make healthy fun. For instance, you could place a delicious lentil burger on a bed of lettuce and dress it up with alfalfa sprouts hair, mustard dotted eyes, a mushroom nose and cherry tomato lips.

Children never have to know they are eating a full spectrum of nutrients and minerals! If it tastes good, which this does, they will gobble it up.

Another thing regarding children, unless they are allergic to certain foods, you shouldn't lament over the fact you cannot always control what they eat outside of the home. It is just not worth the headache. Simply provide nutritious meals in your home as a great start. Also, encourage a daily routine consisting of some form of recreational exercise the whole family can engage in.

I saw this quip written somewhere and found it quite amusing, yet true.

Patient: The problem is obesity runs in my family.

Doctor: The problem is no one runs in your family.

Terri Eileen Liggins

Chapter 7
Breaking the Emotional Ties

Making this transition a successful one is really all about turning off the emotion switch in our brain and turning on the intellect and consciousness switch. I know, I know, I make it sound like it is just as simple as flipping on/off a light switch. Perhaps not initially, but once you have a handle on the emotional connection with food, then the work can begin—but not until then.

Most people don't know, or just don't want to admit it, but they are emotionally ADDICTED to their food—sometimes to the point of insane craziness. Think I'm exaggerating? Consider this. Remember when the makers of Hostess Twinkies® announced they were discontinuing their cream-filled snack? People went ballistic rushing to buy up every box of that cancer-causing stuff. Many even protested the demise of that "golden sponge cake," as they call it. Case closed!

Really, people? A Twinkie is not even real food! It is the farthest as you can get from a healthy snack and people are feeding this to their children on a daily basis. I should know. I ate them almost daily when I was a child, looking forward to seeing that yellow spongy treat as I whipped open my lunchbox. If not that, then there would be a chocolate Hostess® Ho Hos, Ding Dongs or Cupcakes accompanying that bologna and mayo sandwich.

There are enough artificial flavorings and additives in that one snack to do serious damage to a person's organs with consistent use and yet the makers of it were laughing all the way to the bank with that surge of sales. Now that the news frenzy saved it from the grave, it will probably cost you a little more money to kill yourself with a Twinkie.

I saw this cartoon (below) on social media and could not help but share it. I've said it before and it bears saying again...We have become such a backwards nation, thanks in part to emotional ties to food, hence food addictions.

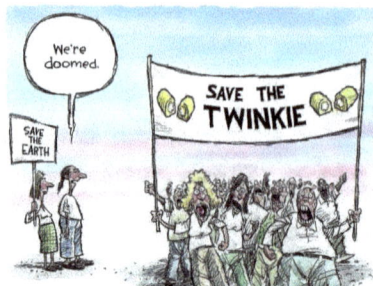

My Journal Entries Regarding Making Conscious Decisions About Food, Not Emotional Ones

September 20, 2012

I realize this is a lonely type of journey I am on. My change in eating style seems to be questioned by some and not taken seriously by others.

Reading an excerpt from Chef Keidi's upcoming book entitled, Living Superfood Research, this resonated so succinctly with me:

> "There is a significant majority within society that considers the idea of solely eating raw foods equivalent to joining some strange religious cult. Yet my experience has shown that one need only sample gourmet living food one time to at least open the mind to the possibility that there could be some value to this "madness." So many have become dumbed-down from eating junk food for so long that they have lost the ability to even conceive the idea of healthy eating and that this should be fundamental. The brain's highest functioning is highly impacted by what we eat. At a certain point the brain can be so damaged by extreme toxicity, that one becomes too "mentally disabled" to protect oneself. When this is a consequence of bad food choices, I refer to the process as "chewicide"; it is far more common than most people want to accept."
> ~Keidi Obi Awadu, aka Chef Keidi

48

April 5, 2013

I am in the picturesque southern hill country of Ohio, visiting one of the most nature-decorated campuses in the U.S., Ohio University (OU). Nestled in Hocking Valley with impressive hills and valleys of green during most of the year and a spectacular show of yellow, orange and red during a too-short fall season, I was fortunate to call this place home for four years back in the late 70's, early 80's. Thirty-two years after I entered those campus gates in Athens, Ohio, my daughter did the same.

Now, I am at my final Mom's Weekend and my daughter's last stage performance of her college theater career. (two sniffs) Beautiful 66 degrees—perfect campus weather. I just dropped her off at her rehearsal, and what was one of the first things I saw? A farmer's market. Yea!

I immediately parked the car and went exploring for goodies. Bought some local honey after the lady selling it assured me their bees were good—meaning not affected by GMOs. Like she can really guarantee that? I'm not sure, but I do know local and raw honey is always ten times better. The indigenous bees producing honey in your own habitat are safest for your body. It works with your immune system, not against it.

I bought a few other goodies there and had a great time exchanging pleasantries. I support local markets whenever possible these days, like I did back in my youthful San Francisco and Chicago days. Back then, I was more conscious of supporting the neighborhood grocers over big chains, shopping for small quantities of food several times a week. Somewhere along my matured and hectic life, I began relying solely on the convenience of those large grocery stores filled with their GMO grown, slime-injected, gluten-ridden, over-priced, processed foods.

Nowadays, even these large chain grocers are hard-pressed to compete against the mega-stores like Wal-Mart, Costco, Sam's Club and the likes. I see people in these stores with their baskets filled to the rim with dangerous toxic food! How did we as a nation come to accept all that? Oh, that's right, I know the answer: Greed on the part of the food industry and laziness on the part of the consumer.

Do you shop at farmer's markets and local mom and pop stores? Whether you are looking to reduce your carbon footprint on this planet, make healthier choices for you and your family, or you're simply on a quest to be supportive of small businesses, kudos to you for doing so!

May 5, 2013

For my daughter's college graduation reception, we prepared a vast living Superfood spread, which included: olive-mushroom pate, bulgar wheat tabouli wraps, mock-chicken salad, guacamole with blue corn chips, hummus, corn salsa, carrot raisin salad, flax crackers, crangerine sauce, marinated greens, organic salad with honey-mustard dressing, chocolate caramel desert, cucumber-lemon water, couscous tabouli, and some things that I probably cannot remember.

The feast was enjoyed by nearly all the 40 or so who attended. I have to say "nearly" because you know there is always someone among us who are just going to refuse to eat healthy no matter what! In fact, it caused some family members to act rather mean-spirited with rude comments here and there.

It's amazing how people approach your table of raw cuisine as though they are being asked to eat a platter of cockroaches or something! There is a real spirit of defiance towards this type of eating. All because they haven't broken *their* emotional tie with food—food that is literally killing them.

The ironic thing is they are turning down REAL food in order to keep eating their FAKE food. Fighting against life to invite death? I will continue to pray for those who remain in the dark about the dangers of processed, fake food to their health.

Chapter 8
Investing in Self

May of 2010. As I sat on the edge of the reclined table in that dead-silent, sterile examination room–thin hospital gown barely shielding my body from the room's rudely cool temperature–one question occupied the entire space in my mind. Earlier that morning, that same space swarmed with a myriad of thoughts of a whole different matter: daily affirmations, end of school year activities and dozens of to-do list items.

The big question

Now, though, one question reverberated there, *"How did his happen?"*

Moments earlier, following a supposed routine mammogram, the physician stepped into this same room to share the results of my x-rays. I heard, *"... found a mass in your breast. Need to do an ultrasound..."* before my mind wandered thousands of miles away. He left the room as abruptly as he came. There I sat—me and this question of mine.

Hearing those words spoken by the doctor was not half as bad as the fact that I was hearing them alone. So, believe it or not, my resounding question *"How did this happen?"* was not referring to *"How did this lump form in my breast?"*

No, no, no. Having been divorced since 2008, the more accurate, emotional translation was, *"How did it come to the fact that I'm dealing with this issue alone?"* No partner to hold my hand through it all; no strong hug accompanied by the assurance that it will all be fine.

Terri Eileen Liggins

We, women

I speak to women all the time in this same situation: single and left to deal with crucial life-altering decisions on their own. That is, if there's even time to deal with their crisis while helping everyone else with theirs.

Usually, women, from this group of 74 million American baby boomers, are the caregivers for aging parents and simultaneously for children in the home. Because of this, the busyness of the day does not allow them to properly attend to their health. Well, let me rephrase that. Women have not been properly taught/guided/programmed to attend to their health first and foremost. Unfortunately, those who *have* mastered this art risk being labeled self-centered or, heaven forbid, un-nurturing.

With today's statistics showing 1 in every 3 baby boomer now single (a combination of divorced and never-married 50 and 60 year-olds),[11] more women than ever before are challenged to do more and be more. Doing more and being more is a tall order when health issues get in the way. I should know.

Upon suffering a heart attack at age 40, and being on 15 different medications over the course of six months thereafter, I was not well enough to be of great assistance to my then-husband or a Super-Mom to my two elementary-age children. I was, however, blessed in that the heart attack and sarcoidosis were warnings to get my priorities straight, instead of situations that abruptly ended my life.

To clarify that statement I just made, I am not saying I was blessed to have been stricken with these illnesses. I hear people state that kind of weirdness all the time: *"God made me ill to get my attention." "God brought these trials on me to teach me a lesson."* What does that mean? I don't buy that ONE BIT! If your god is such a loving god, why would He do that?

Would a loving earthly parent put their child's hand on a stove's lit burner to teach them not to touch the stove? Of course not! Then, why would our

---

[11] Taking cues from "The Golden Girls," more baby boomers are building a future together. PBS News Hour (2014).
Retrieved from: www.pbs.org/newshour/bb/baby-boomers-take-cues-from-golden-girls on May 30, 2017.

heavenly Father, with so much more love for us than an earthly parent, do that? In fact, the Bible says His house is not divided. So, if He's injuring you, then making you well again, that sounds pretty divided to me.

Must own up

So maybe *your* god would do that, but I have a hard time believing mine would. It doesn't make logical sense. Therefore, in my opinion, God didn't make you sick; YOU made you sick. You are never going to change your habits in order to get well and stay well until you first own that truth.

Owning the truth must be the first step in investing in you. Investing in you is the only way to declare victory over sickness and disease.

What truth did *I* have to own up to? That, ten years after my first health crisis and seven years after I had begun to make healthier choices (cutting out red meats, sugar and carbs), I was still dealing with health issues— another major one at that. Possible breast cancer. Therefore, whatever I was doing to get well wasn't enough.

Test results

I went in for a biopsy of that lumpy breast a couple weeks later. Thank goodness the results were benign. Had it been otherwise, I shudder to think what treatments I would've opted for. Not having the knowledge that I have now of food being God's perfect medicine—yes even for cancer—I just may have opted for horrible alternatives that too often women are bamboozled into. I don't mean to sound harsh or judgmental of those who have chosen that route, but again, I'm just owning the truth for *me*.

My actual medical report from that procedure[12] is a staunch reminder to me and hopefully a warning to others about the dangerous consequence of not investing in your health preventatively by making good health practices a priority. The bad foods that I ate, my lack of regular exercise, my bad sleeping habits and my high levels of stress all contributed to this grouping of cysts.

This procedure was painful—more mentally than physically. Save yourself from that.

---

[12] See Appendix A. Page 95. Figure 2.

By the way, what *was* physically painful about this procedure (I remember it like it was yesterday) was that very soon after putting this 22-gauge needle in my breast to extract the mass, they sent me through another mammogram. Seriously? At the very place where my breast is still sore, you're going to smash it to smithereens? I wanted to scream. They said they had to make sure they got it all. I am convinced it had to be a man who developed that procedure and the equipment.

We must invest fully in the notion that food is nature's most powerful and effective medicine. Looking to drop some pounds the safe and permanent way? Whole, plant-based food is the answer. Looking to prevent sickness and disease? Whole, plant-based food is the answer. Looking to reverse a bad report by the doctor—allergies, auto-immune disorders, high blood pressures, diabetes, cancers, and such? Whole, plant-based food is the answer. Invest in it today; invest in you for a lifetime.

My Journal Entries Regarding Investing in Food for Overall Wellbeing and Weight Loss

October 6, 2012

I'm now learning new things about the chemical aspect of foods. For instance, natural hygienists have been telling people for years that fruit doesn't combine well with other foods. They contain simple sugars requiring no digestion. Those sugars do not stay long in your stomach, which is why fruit is so good for you to eat. Your body turns the fructose to fuel and eliminates the rest.

On the other hand, foods rich in fat, protein, and starch, stay in your stomach for a long time because they require more digestive work. So, if you eat fruit right after a full meal, its sugar will remain for too long in the stomach along with the other stuff and will ferment. That is why it is recommended fruit be eaten alone and not with other foods. For similar reasons, it is recommended that you eat melons alone and avoid mixing acid fruits with sweet fruits such as bananas.

November 19, 2012

Living super foods was put to the test as not only a natural source of medicinal properties to ward off illnesses and disease, but also a way to stay alive in the wake of trauma. After living a vegetarian lifestyle for about 30 years, Chef Keidi Awadu advanced up several rungs on the food hierarchy ladder. His dietary regimen since 2009 has consisted of a full spectrum of raw, hyper nutritional meals called super foods, along with seasonal detoxification fasts.

Chef Keidi is alive and well today but was struck by a drunk driver on a major street in Los Angeles two days ago. The young drunk female swerved towards the curb while he was placing some items into the back of his parked vehicle. He never saw it coming; was hit from behind; knocked unconscious; and woke up with a crowd of people standing over him as paramedics placed him in the ambulance.

Even though he was between his car and the speeding (according to witnesses) car; even though his car was totaled in the process; and even though he suffered 19 separate injuries; Chef Keidi did not endure one single broken bone! Now, that is a miracle from above and a testament to the importance of keeping your body in tip top shape to handle any catastrophic impact that comes your way!

Staying true to his character, he joked through his pain in the trauma unit, refused meds and refused to stay there overnight. Once home, he did not take a single prescribed pill throughout his entire three-month healing period— not even an aspirin!

Chef Keidi only engaged in holistic muscle-stimulating treatments, natural supplements and herbs. Pain throughout his entire body was very intense at times. He suffered through body temperatures of up to 103 degrees most of the time as well, which is a sign the body is fighting off infection. Overall, his recovery time was shorter than if he consumed conventional medicine that only dulls the pain and inhibits the healing process.

His ordeal is also a true testament to the importance of celebrating the people in our lives EVERY DAY, not just on their birthdays or certain holidays. With this being the Thanksgiving holiday season, it is a great time to be ever so mindful of just how fragile life is. Take an extra moment to appreciate friends, family, co-workers, acquaintances and loved ones. Not only is our time on earth precious but sometimes it's preciously short.

February 3, 2013

One quite easy way to help beat the urge to go back to unhealthy snacking is to keep a large amount of fresh fruit and veggies in your home.

Except right before shopping day, when our fruit basket is bare, you will always find bananas, tangerines, oranges, apples, grapefruit and various melons gracing our dining table. Other fruit generally kept in the house are strawberries, lemons, limes, raisins and sometimes dehydrated apricots and cranberries.

Grocery shopping with a different perspective is a major step towards investing in your family's health. Not just for today but for generations to come!

February 22, 2013

This week was my six-month anniversary of becoming a rawtarian! During this time, 99% of the foods I have eaten have contained live enzymes instead of saturated fats, toxins and chemicals. I eat more now than before, yet my weight is decreasing! My major health issues have cleared, as well!

The bonus to eating healthy has been this effortless weight loss. I say effortless, because I don't exercise regularly. I am still attempting to fit that in my crazy and sedentary writing schedule.

Right now, I weigh 127 pounds—just three pounds away from the weight I was in my twenties! Yea! Can I do it? Can I do it? Can I drop those last five pounds that I'm shooting for? If only I can stick with an exercise program to tone up my muscles, this 54-year-old body would be hot! Seriously.

Who would like to join me in this journey back to our mid-20's weight? For most of us women, that means back to our pre-childbearing weight. Come on; if I can do this, you can, too!

By the way, before now, I had always been too embarrassed to share this very personal information. I hid my excess weight well with my clothes. Most people who tried to guess it, usually came in much lower. Just know that sharing my weight publicly in this book is a very big deal. So, consider yourself privileged. (Smile.) And to think when I first started on this journey, the scale registered me at 147 pounds. (Yikes! I'm really getting bold revealing such personal information.)

August 9, 2013

Down from a size 8 dress to a size 2 in just one year. Not bad. I've taken in the seams of my clothes as much as I can and I CAN'TS no more (in my best Popeye voice)! Time to purge the closet and buy new clothes since almost everything in there makes me look frumpy. Subconsciously I thought I would return to some of those clothes. But nope, I am NOT going back, if I have anything to do with it—and by golly, I have EVERYTHING to do with it!

A couple friends who had not seen me in years asked to see a photo of the new me. I hadn't been satisfied enough with my body to post an "after" photos. I needed to exercise first to tone up; however, my daily work schedule would usually interfere with any consistency in exercising. (That is my excuse and I'm sticking to it!)

Recently, I started doing stomach crunches and planks and within a short period of time got up to 120 crunches per day and 75-second planks. Finally, I decided it was time for a photo of me.

I had a favorite size 4 red dress I kept in my closet for many years, just waiting for the chance to wear it. I had gotten it from my sister and was never quite able to zip it all the way up. Periodically, I'd try it on with no success; vowing each time to give up and give it away. An inner voice would quickly say, "Naw, hold on to it."

Well, today I am finally putting on that coveted size 4 dress. Guess what? Now, it is slightly *too big* for me!

Terri Eileen Liggins

Chapter 9
Embracing Detoxification

In extracting information from my journal pages about the first three fasts I performed during my first year of eating raw, it became apparent to me just how extensive the information was. I didn't want to get too detailed in explaining everything because detox cleansing works best when it is custom designed to your body's needs. Therefore, I didn't want you to read about what I had done and what my results were thinking that you would have to do that too, or that you would experience what I experienced.

You can use my detox fast as a guide only (just as I used Chef Keidi's), but trial and error is the best method for determining what will bring you optimal results. That comes from seeing how your body reacts to each stage of the fast. By the time you have done three or so fasts, you'll know what method "moves" you.

What is it?

Detoxification, in a nutshell, is removing impurities from your bloodstream by various methods involving food elimination, juices or supplements.

Why do it?

In the body's natural and healthy cleansing process, toxins, parasites, chemicals, free radicals and such are eliminated through the liver, kidneys, intestines, lungs, lymph and skin. However, in an unhealthy body—one that has never been cleansed—this process gets all gummed up and impurities aren't being properly filtered. When this occurs, almost every cell in your body is adversely affected. Detoxing fixes all that.

Detoxifying the body is vitally important to help prevent abnormal cell function. Cells can become abnormal or mutated from exposure to ionzing radiation or 'mistakes' in cell division which changes the chemical properties of genetic materials. The mutated cell can divide uncontrollably, and form clusters called tumors. These tumors are what we then call cancer.

When a person is taking in more calories than they are burning, the result will be stored body fat. The same is true with toxins. When the intake of toxins is greater than the amount that is being removed through detoxification, a person suffers from toxic overload. If a person is overweight, you instantly know they are storing up a massive amount of toxins. However, even individuals at a normal weight are harboring loads of bad gut bacteria and other harmful free radicals in their bodies if they never detox. Bottom line, toxins in the body is the source of disease. Cleansing the body of these toxins will at least reduce their symptoms, if not cure it.

Some of the ways we introduce toxins into our body's cells on a daily basis:

1. Inhaling air pollution
2. Using cleaning solutions with formaldehyde and ammonia
3. Wearing clothes saturated with chemical fabric softeners
4. Drinking water laced with chlorine
5. Using shampoos, deodorants, mouthwashes, and toothpastes loaded with a multitude of chemicals
6. Eating loads of foods containing a myriad of chemicals, additives and unpronounceable names like sodium stearoyl-2-lactylate, monoglycerides and L-Cysteine hydrochloride

Some of the ways a detox program restores the body's natural cleansing process:

1. Resting the organs through fasting
2. Stimulating the liver to drive toxins from the body
3. Promoting elimination through the intestines, kidneys and skin
4. Improving circulation of the blood
5. Refueling the body with healthy nutrients

Who should do it?

Basically, everyone should detox at least twice a year to maintain good health. Even children can cleanse using a mild method. You should especially do a body cleanse if you suffer from any of these or other health issues:

1. Diabetes
2. High blood pressure
3. Ulcers
4. Blood diseases like sickle cell anemia

Even if a person is not suffering from disease or illness, they still need to do a detox at least twice a year, if they:

1. live in the city
2. eat a lot of meat
3. eat chemically processed foods
4. eat pesticide-contaminated vegetables
5. eat food that contains white flour and white sugar
6. take prescription drugs
7. are regularly stressed out

Juice fasting

Before I get into the heavy-duty detoxing, let me share that using juices as a form of detoxing is a great idea. It may be much easier for the novice as well. A juice fast helps to break up the sticky mucus in us. It allows you to target specific body systems: kidneys, blood vessels, blood, immune system, and nervous system. Be sure to drink the juice immediately after making it so the nutrients are not lost through oxidation.

Here are a few juices and their attributes. Without giving specific credit, just know that the information comes from simply Googling around the Internet. So, head to the internet and find lots of juicing variations like these to jumpstart your healthier lifestyle:

61

Watermelon – Among the many minerals in this wonder-fruit are lycopene, a powerful antioxidant, known to protect your cardiovascular system from free radical damage, and citru-line, an amino acid that can be converted in your body into arginine, an essential amino acid for improving blood flow and relaxing blood vessels. Its benefits are too numerous to mention them all here, but I must share that watermelon is a great diuretic for the kidneys, flushing out ammonia and uric acid. Be sure to buy your watermelons with the seeds if using the juice for kidney cleansing, as the seeds offer the highest cleansing effect.

Cabbage – Cabbage juice is a traditional treatment for healing ulcers, as it strengthens the mucosal linings of the gastrointestinal tract. Patients have been able to heal their ulcers within 10 days by drinking just a liter of cabbage juice daily. Drinking this juice also creates a significant reduction in blood levels of low-density lipoprotein, the so-called bad cholesterol.

Apple/pear – Apples and pears contain fructose. Besides this sugar giving both these fruits their sweet taste, fructose metabolizes slower than sucrose and does not create a spike in blood sugar levels in the way sucrose does. An apple/pear juice is great for digestion. It has vitamin C, essential for a healthy immune system and a phytochemical called quercetin, for anti-inflammatory functioning. This juice is best when consumed right before going to bed.

Carrot/apple/celery – A combination of carrots, apples and celery put through a juicer offers a potassium and sodium ratio (mainly due to the celery) that effectively stimulates urine and helps to remove excess water and uric acid from the kidneys. This juice is also great for weight loss, aiding in sleep and getting rid of headaches, just to name a few benefits.

Detox fasting

Whether you do a simple juice fast, or a detox program consisting of various phases (as shared in my journal entries), the bottom line is, the human body is an amazing cluster of energy making up the finest temple in the known universe. At some point, we must say "enough is enough" of our efforts to wreck it. We must take control over habits that are contrary to optimum health and vitality; habits that lead to sickness, disease, a weakened immune system, and ultimately premature death.

Besides cleansing the body's organs, the rewards for detoxing are simply awesome! They include heightened intuition, increased clairvoyance, rapid weight loss, increased energy, heightened spiritual awareness and appreciation of the many blessings that fill our lives. There is also the reward of money saved each week from what you would've been spending on food.

On December 21, 2012, I started my first ever detoxification fast. It was the first day of winter. I stayed on it for seven days, through December 27. Today, I continue the habit of beginning my fast the first day of each new season: Winter Solstice, Spring Equinox, Summer Solstice and Autumn Equinox.

The Winter Solstice fast overlaps the Christmas holiday. That meant no Christmas dinner for me as a novice at this fasting thing. I had been raw for only four months; yet I was okay with no holiday meal. After all, I looked at this journey as not a diet that I can jump off and back on again. No, no, no! Its purpose was a lifestyle change. One must never mistake one for the other.

Dieting is counterproductive. Dieting is dangerous because of the typical yo-yo mindset of eating healthy for a while, then going back to eating things that are bad. While on the other hand, a committed lifestyle change for the better is just that, a lifestyle. And guess what? Life doesn't allow for time-off from everything. I believe that is called dying.

I was already on that dying route when I discovered life again and jumped that train transporting me to a period of senior years filled with meds and pain. Why would I go back to that simply because tradition tells me I need to eat a dinner full of toxic ingredients?

Both my children were home from college for that Christmas holiday in 2012. I felt a little bad they would not get a huge, home-cooked traditional spread, complete with all the trimmings. However, why should I feel bad about them *not* getting to eat horribly dangerous food, right? I don't.

However, I knew they weren't ready for this lifestyle change, even being privy to credible information through me. They were young adults with minds of their own. Children have an innate tendency to not want to do as you say because after all, you are *just* their parent. Juxtaposed is the notion that they will, however, tend to do as you *do*! Having people watch what you do (no matter what it is in life), and showing them the outcome that follows, is a more guaranteed method of bringing about action. That is where good parenting prevails.

Fortunately for my children, on that Christmas day, my cousin who lived in town invited them to a traditional feast with her daughter-in-law's family. They went and I stayed home to celebrate the holiday by honoring my body with prune juice and herbal supplements.

I am happy to report that as of the printing of this book, both my children are fully committed raw vegans. (Yea!) My son became a health advocate while in college. He was very instrumental in his upperclassman, 45-student, co-ed house adopting raw vegan meals as part of their daily menu created by their house chef. Soon after her college graduation, my daughter followed in my footsteps of an all-round healthy lifestyle. Aside from her food, she uses only organic or natural personal care products and home cleaning products. She has been very vocal in sharing this lifestyle with her friends, family, colleagues, and clients.

My Journal Entries Regarding My Detoxification Fasts

WINTER SOLSTICE

December 21, 2012 – Day One – starting weight: 139.8
48-hour water-only phase

This is my first ever detox. I started off today with water only now and for the next 48 hours.

This is the first day of Winter, first day of the Winter Solstice. A lot of firsts going on here. Winter Solstice means the sun's elevation with respect to the North Pole is at its most negative value since this same time last year and the elevation with respect to the South Pole is at its greatest value. Also, during this time, the hemisphere experiences its longest night and shortest day.

I'm supposed to weigh myself every morning after elimination. This will definitely form a new habit as I hadn't owned a scale in years. Hated what it showed me; was going to the doctor often enough that I figured the weigh-ins there were plenty. However, I am learning that one of the ways to help me manage my weight is to SEE it; and often. Ugh! So, I bought a scale. Okay, here it goes. I'm actually going to start writing down my weight every day.

The last doctor visit I had back in August of this year (before I went raw), I weighed a whopping 147 pounds! That was even more than I weighed at nine months pregnant! Today, at the start of this detox and after going raw four months ago, I'm down about seven pounds, weighing 139.8 pounds. Still too heavy, but that weight loss was without any exercising.

December 22, 2012 – Day Two – starting weight: 137.2
48-hour water-only phase

Drank 80 ounces of water today. Down almost two pounds! Other than the fact that I'm dreaming of dehydrated kale chips and yam chips (yum, yum), I'm doing great! Feel great; look great! Not tired. I am pushing past the stomach growls. I just have to wrap my mind around the next phase.

December 23, 2012 – Day Three – starting weight: 135.2
Colon/ parasite cleanse phase

After my first glass of water for the day, herbal laxatives (two Cascara Sagrada capsules) and a parasite cleanse supplement (two CKLS capsules) is all I took today—three times, eight hours apart. Along with drinking lots of water, I am drinking prune juice while taking the herbal laxative tablets.

December 24, 2012 – Day Four – starting weight: 134.8
Colon/ parasite cleanse phase

This is the 4th day of no food and it is becoming tough. Repeat capsules from yesterday. Bowels really moved well.

By late day, I became a wimp, hit a brick wall with my stamina. I whined and reasoned with my mind about how a teeny bit of food would be ok. So, I broke down and ate just a tiny bit of carrot raisin salad.

I am not giving in to this, just needed a little substance. Or at least I let my flesh convince my Spirit Man that I needed that food. Oh well, enough of shaming myself; I am moving forward. For the rest of the journey, I got it together.

December 25, 2012 – Day Five – starting weight: 133.2
Chelation therapy phase

Chelation is a process of using supplements to bind the heavy metals, minerals and toxins in your body, grab them and eliminate them. To do this, once every couple of hours I took a teaspoon of Bentonite Clay along with one EDTA (calcium disodium) capsule.

Today is Christmas, symbolizing to Christians God's greatest gift: His Son. His Son symbolizes new birth and everlasting life. Well, today, I'm giving a gift back to God: the "bestest" most healthiest me possible to exist in this temporary temple called my body. Being the best me allows me to successfully run this race called humanity long enough and focused enough to come into full fruition with my purpose here on this earth.

Finding my purpose and then operating in that purpose throughout the remainder of my journey on this earth is my obligation. Optimal health and wealth is my reward to myself while fulfilling that obligation. That is why, even though it's Christmas, I'm not partaking of a traditional Christmas dinner—that would go against my reward. I'm glad my children were able to go with my cousin to her daughter-in-law's for dinner. As for me and my body, we will honor the holiday with a clean body.

December 26, 2012 – Day Six – starting weight: 131.2
Chelation therapy phase

Day 6 of my detox and the second day of the chelation therapy. I simply repeated yesterday's routine, forgetting a couple doses throughout the day.

Today, I came across a Facebook posting about OU's [Ohio University, Athens, Ohio] favorite food places. You may agree that college life offers some of the fondest food memories one could ever have. This is mainly because of the emotional attachments we have to certain foods due to the friendships built while consuming that stuff. Just like the emotional times to a traditional Thanksgiving or Christmas dinner.

My emotional ties would be with: *The Hole in the Wall* sub shop, *Miller's Chicken* take-out restaurant, (still there after 30+ years and still a favorite of alums when back on campus for reunions), gyros from *Souvlaki's Mediterranean Gardens* (another one of Athens' proud and oldest eatery), the 2:00 am visits to *The Bagel Buggy* up town for strawberry bagels with cream cheese, and the list goes on. I can still taste them all!

What I am learning throughout this fast is that when you "try," chances are you'll falter; when you "do" and do it with mustard seed faith and a pound of determination, you will no doubt find out just how strong your mind is over your flesh. After all, if you can't overcome a hamburger, how are you going to conquer major demons in your life?"

I went into this fast just "trying" it and on the 4th day of no food it became tough. I whined and reasoned with my mind about how a teeny bit of food would be ok. I ate just a few morsels of raw super foods but that's ok, I didn't quit and now at day six, I'm doing great.

December 27, 2012 – Day Seven – starting weight: 130.2

This is Day 7 of my detox. I feel great! Down nine pounds. Yea! Could've been more if I'd been exercising like I knew I was supposed to. I ended my fast here.

Between my time spent in LA, a sprang or bruised tendon in my foot during my recent house move, picking kids up from airport, and the gym's holiday schedule, it has been two months since going to my hot Pilates class. UGH!

Nonetheless, I'm ecstatic about the nine pounds gone and looking to "off" many more pounds over the months to come. I intended to do a two-week detox fast but it ended up being only seven days. Oh well, at least I did it! Congratulations, me!

SPRING EQUINOX

March 20 – 24, 2013
A repeat of my Winter Solstice detox. Starting weight: 132.8. Ending weight: 125

Time for my Spring Equinox detoxification fast! Generally, the length of time to stay on this fast is 7, 14, or 28 days—whichever one you can handle. Obviously, for optimum results, it is suggested to go all 28 days.

This time around, I only did five days, last time was seven. If you were to ask me why I haven't fasted for longer periods of time, I would have to admit I don't have a specific reason other than I just haven't committed myself to doing so. To begin a fast, let alone complete one successfully, it requires one's full mental capacity. I found that out rather quickly in December 2012.

At the time I started my first detox fast ever, I didn't do all my homework about detoxing, nor did I ask all the right questions of Chef Keidi who had introduced me to the practice of detoxing. By day two, I was so hungry that I swore I wasn't going to make it! By day three Chef Keidi got so tired of hearing me whine that he told me I could have a handful of peanuts.

Basically, I was defeated before I even started because I didn't settle the matter in my mind first. However, once I started seeing the results—one to two pounds per day of weight dropping off—I was sold on the process. More important than just the weight loss, knowing my bowels were pushing out all those toxins was quite exciting for me. That made it possible to finish out the seven days.

Like before, there were four stages to my detox program: first the water fast; next the colon cleanse and parasite cleanse (I combine these two phases since I shorten my whole detox period down to seven days; otherwise, I would give them each two separate days); and finally, chelation therapy. After that, I targeted some organs by drinking 10 ounces of virgin olive oil straight. No break until the glass is empty or else you could gag on it and that would not be pleasant. I chased it with 100% organic lemon juice and then stayed close to home, if you know what I mean.

This process cleanses the gall bladder and liver and can likely release gall stones with your stool. I must admit, *I* didn't see any signs of stones (supposedly emerald in color) like others have told me they experienced.

SUMMER SOLSTICE

June 21 – 27, 2013
A repeat of my Winter Solstice detox. Starting weight: 127. Ending weight: 120

This time, I went seven days again like with the Winter Solstice. Each time I perform my detox, there are some slight variations. You must listen to your body and give it what it needs and can handle. Don't worry; it will let you know exactly what that is.

As I mentioned before, following the chelation therapy I target certain organs by drinking olive oil to help move all those toxins and gall stones right out of your body. This is the last part of the detox fast. It is by far the most dreaded part for me. Ten ounces of olive oil down the hatch chased by a little bit of freshly squeezed lemon juice.

The last time, as well as this time, I videotaped myself drinking that and posted it up on YouTube. I thought this time around would be easier to manage. Not quite the case, although I still drank it all just like before. Some of my viewers said they were cringing while watching me chug it down. How funny.

Yes, it is a slightly unpleasant procedure. However, I still give it a thumbs-up when it comes to giving your body a periodic cleansing from all the damage done to it from the toxins we inhale from the air and those we ingest.

Terri Eileen Liggins

FALL EQUINOX FAST

September 22 – 30, 2013
A repeat of my Winter Solstice detox. Starting weight: 124.4. Ending weight: 119

This is my fourth time doing this detox fast. Seven days again. I didn't lose as many pounds this time as I anticipated because we conducted a food demo on the sixth day of the fast and I did consume several small amounts of the Superfood dishes Chef Keidi prepared. As I assist in these demos as the sous chef, I am tasting the foods from time to time. Not good in the middle of my fast, but oh well, I still finished it out on that seventh day.

I cannot stress enough to people that it is important to find out what works for them when doing a detox fast. Even though I attempt to develop a pattern with my detoxing, each time is different and that is perfectly okay. I am proud of myself for continuing on this path of periodically cleansing my body all the way down to my cells, even more so than with my everyday practice of eating clean.

Part III

My Meals

Chapter 10
Stuff I Eat

"So, what exactly do you eat?" With scrunched up nose and one eye closed, the inquirer is prepared to hear something like: bitter wheatgrass juice along with carrots and celery sticks. I've been asked that question so many times it only made sense to devote an entire chapter to this topic.

Before I talk about the specifics of what I eat, I must reiterate how important it is to focus on the WHY of eating healthy. Even if you haven't figured out the why by this 10th chapter, have no fear, it will all make sense at some point—sooner for some than others. The important thing is that we all get there!

Focusing on the why of eating healthy gives you the tenacity to persevere when the going gets tough. When no one else around you is eating this way; when you don't have time to prepare the meals; and when the cost of buying healthy food seems way too high, those are the tough times you must push through.

Well, you know what? Chances are, very few people around you, if any, *are* maintaining a raw, plant-based food regimen. Yes, this food *does* take a little more time to prepare, as there is no poke-a-pouch-and-microwave-it activity allowed. But isn't your good health worth that extra time? Finally, yes, the organic ingredients *do* tend to cost a little more at the grocery store, but I can guarantee you being sick costs even more. That, I know first-hand.

Besides, it's not that fruits and vegetables, in and of themselves are expensive. *Organic* fruits, vegetables, and *organic* veggie drinks are expensive. So, don't fall for that "only buy organic" spiel. Sure, organic is best, but work with what you can afford. As long as you wash the fruit and veggies really well (organic and non-organic), you'll be fine. The way I see it, a little dirty greens is still a lot better to your bloodstream than artery-clogging red meat.

In addition to getting rid of diseases or illnesses, one of the big WHYs people have for eating healthy is to look better. Is it okay to focus so much on improving your outer appearance? Absolutely! As long as you do it with a healthy, positive mindset and not in some vain attempt to mask deeper issues that you are not allowing yourself to be freed from. Ex: Dieting excessively in a non-nutritious manner just to flaunt your slim body revengefully in front of an ex-boyfriend.

Self-confidence goes hand in hand with that notion of looking healthy. I believe one begets the other. Let's face it; it's hard to have self-confidence when you're not feeling your best. It is hard to feel your best when you're not looking your best and your body is chugging along in a sluggish fashion. On the contrary, when you are feeling great from the inside out, exerting high energy with positive vibrations and all, self-confidence automatically soars!

To me, this health journey is all about confidence building. It's about learning to love everything about your body—that which you can change as well as that which you cannot. Body shaming, which I had been guilty of doing to MYSELF for way too long, does anything BUT build self-confidence.

So, say good-bye to body shaming through negative inner judgment and criticism. Say hello to confidence through self-love and high esteem! After all, it's next to impossible to accomplish any of your life goals without self-confidence.

Now, back to the food…

Most people, upon tasting our living superfood meals, love them. However, every once in a while, we'll have a guest at dinner who will put a heaping amount of something on their plate only to later scoop half of it into the trash. Ouch! That is a lot of money down the drain!

No doubt, they thought the food would taste like one thing, but it tasted totally different. It may have been a flavor or texture their taste buds weren't prepared for. Believe it or not, the dislike is usually simply because the food is cold, not hot. Too often we have seen that one. A person's brain has a hard time grasping that one difference. Thank goodness most people can get past that. Once they do, they can begin to love the new flavorful freshness they are experiencing.

So, here are three easy steps to remember when trying raw cuisine for the first time:

1. Know that there is nothing to be afraid! It is all REAL food making it onto your plate from God's green earth, in a purer form.

2. Because it's not everyone's cup of tea, start off by putting just a tiny bit on your plate. Trust me, that won't insult the chef; whereas, throwing away food that was so specifically prepared *will* insult him or her.

3. Enjoy the fact that, with each delicious bite, trillions of cells in your body are being happily nourished; thereby restoring each organ to its proper function, allowing you to once again skip, jump and run!

During my first year of going raw, I journaled a lot about what I was eating and how simple or difficult it was to prepare. I'm happy to share that experience with you to help you see "it's nothing but a thang!" In some of the entries, I reference Appendix B where you can find a photo of what my meal looks like.

With raw meals, you will notice the colorfulness of the food. Rule of thumb: The more colorful your plate, the healthier it is. So, ditch the unhealthy, brown and white, meat and potatoes kind of meal for those vibrant colors representing health and wellness!

Terri Eileen Liggins

My Journal Entries Regarding the New Foods Introduced to Me

September 1, 2012

Happy Labor Day! I'm spending it in Los Angeles tasting a plate of Chef Keidi's full spectrum hyper nutrition "Living Superfood" for the first time. Delicious and so very filling! Much different than the one or two items from his recipe book I had been making over and over at home.

Keidi even had me preparing a goji berry juice. I don't think I ever even heard of goji berries before now. They are classified as a super food. They are also around $12.99 a pound. Yikes!

Excellent taste—gotta make this again! It is a rather expensive drink, but hey, I'm worth it, right?

Besides, as with most things on this new health journey, I'm learning to put it all into perspective. For example, people don't flinch at all when paying anywhere from $4.25 to $8.25 per drink at a bar, right? Even paying much more for the real high-grade stuff. Spending a lot of money putting sugary toxins in their precious body.

However, if a healthy drink like this cost $4 or $5 dollars—with ingredients PROVEN to heal you—the first thing people want to do is complain that it's too expensive to eat healthy. Hmm. I've come to the conclusion that we are a real funny and backwards society.

September 2, 2012

Labor Day weekend continues. Another living super foods dinner. This yummy meal full of nutrients, proteins and live enzymes is helping to protect me against heart disease.

About 49% of all Americans are flirting with the risk factors of heart (cardiovascular) disease, by either not caring about, or not being knowledgeable of its risk factors. They put themselves at a higher risk by choices like obesity, poor diet, physical inactivity and excessive alcohol use.[13]

One in four deaths that occur in the U.S. each year is due to cardiovascular disease—that's 600,000 people.[14] Unfortunately, these statistics will repeat year after year, and they don't have to!

I am deciding today that I will avoid being a statistic of the much-overlooked phenomenon of malnutrition and dehydration. Those two words drum up the image of an anorexic-looking, shriveled up person when that is not at all the case. Now that I learned a thing or two, I know that obesity is a form of malnutrition. It is causing diseases galore, killing its victims in the process.

The meal I had today consisted of sesame sunflower bread; carrot raisin salad; zucchini spaghetti with marinara sauce; nut balls; pear-apple sauce; kale pesto; and cut vegetables (lettuce, tomato and cucumber). On the side are roasted barley ice tea and almond yogurt with pineapples.[15]

September 7, 2012

I did it! I did it! It may not be one of Chef Keidi's magnificent 10-item meals, but I made "mock" chicken salad all by myself. No cooking, no can opening, no meat. It is good and is good for me. Off with another two pounds, also. Yea!

Now, I have mastered about four meals. Hmm, what shall I try next?

It's all about taking baby steps—doing what I can the best way I know how, without beating myself up in the process. It's been almost a month since I decided to go raw. Even though I've eaten one or two processed crackers or pretzels here and there, as well as some sushi, I don't consider that having fallen off the bandwagon. I intend to never fully leave the bandwagon; even

---

[13] Center for Disease Control and Prevention. (2011) *Million Hearts: strategies to reduce the prevalence of leading cardiovascular disease risk factors.* United States. MMWR2011;60(36):1248–51

[14] Murphy SL, Xu JQ, Kochanek KD. (2013) *Deaths: Final data for 2010.* National Vital Statistics Report;61(4) Retrieved Jan 2014 from www.cdc.gov/nchs/data/nvsr/nvsr61/nvsr61_04.pdf

[15] Appendix B. Page 100. Figure 1.

Terri Eileen Liggins

though, who knows, some variations may possibly be made down through the years.

Note: The recipe for Mock-Chicken is found on page 44 of *Living Superfood Recipes*.

October 8, 2012

Mom nailed it! I enjoyed a delicious raw dinner at home with Mom before heading back to the West Coast in the morning. She made Chef Keidi's own "Spinach Save-My-Life Soup" all by herself. It was delicious!

It has 19 ingredients, so it can seem a bit overwhelming for someone looking at the recipe for the first time. However, it is not so bad after all when you consider the fact that most of those 19 ingredients are just spices.

I showed Mom a trick I use with that recipe to make it easier to prepare. I mix together all the dry ingredients only, which again are mainly spices. I mix four times the amount the recipe calls for. I then scoop that mixture equally into four very small plastic containers or snack baggies, labeling the containers and storing them in the pantry.

That way, whenever I want to make this soup, I just grab a container, dump in the mixture along with the wet ingredients and voilá—the prep time is cut in half. Now, that is how I like it—quick and simple!

Great job, Mom. The Mock-Chicken salad you made was superb, as well!

Note: The recipe for Spinach Save-My-Life Soup is found on page 41 of *Living Superfood Recipes Vol 2*

November 10, 2012

We had a great *Living Superfood* demonstration today at my girlfriend Tamara's house. She has a very nice kitchen with one of the biggest and baddest granite-top islands I've seen (besides in magazines). It is custom made and ten feet long. It was just the perfect space for Chef Keidi to prepare a lot of dishes for six of us to sample. We also enjoyed some dishes that he prepared in advance. Our meal consisted of mock-chicken salad, flax crackers, carrot raisin salad, kale seaweed salad, dehydrated tomatoes; not-cheese paté, crangerine sauce; chocolate haystacks and yam chips.

Items not pictured included: natural potato chips, nut milk, choco-banana super shake and roasted barley tea.[16]

Whew! Our bellies were completely satisfied with no worries about excessive calories, high sugar or salt intake, and especially no dangerous chemicals and additives. What is not to love about a delicious meal with all of those advantages?

Imagine preparing delicious, healthy gourmet meals in *your* dream kitchen. You deserve such a treat, don't you? I know *I* do, so I am working on both.

December 3, 2012

It's moving day today! In the midst of boxes strewn throughout the new house, we managed to find a few food items to throw together.

Our meal consisted of: mock-chicken, color salad with beets, tomatoes and chocolate haystack. We made a salad dressing from olive oil, hemp protein, Spirulina and some spices.[17]

Lots of black sesame seeds are always good to sprinkle on your food because they are known to be beneficial for strong bones and teeth. White sesame seeds are great for essential fatty acids, amino acids and tryptophan. Since Chef Keidi is still on the mends from that drunk driver plowing him down last month, these super nutrient seeds are greatly needed to recharge all the muscles in his injured legs. Don't *you* also deserve to have *your* super body super charged?

December 12, 2012

Shhh! Don't tell anyone, but I just had fudge for breakfast. Oh, that's right, it's okay for me to eat fudge any time of the day because mine is prepared the LIVE way! This fudge consists of raw coconut butter, raw cacao powder, mesquite powder and organic agave nectar. All raw, all natural, no cooking involved wreaking havoc on your immune system.[18]

---

[16] Appendix B. page 100. Figure 2.

[17] Appendix B. page 100. Figure 3.

[18] Appendix B. page 100. Figure 4.

It is so good and so sweet it could win any dessert contest. More importantly, eating this won't wreak havoc on my immune system, preventing me from fighting off diseases and symptoms associated with this so-called flu season.

I say "so-called" because I am not totally convinced that a virus permeates our communities at a heightened rate *only* during these cold months of the year. What I *am* convinced of is that from Halloween through Valentine's Day, children and adults in America overdose on sugar, high fructose corn syrup, artificial flavors and colors, as well as other junk food due to holiday eating traditions.

Such extreme dietary indulgence in sugar is the greatest cause of immune system malfunction there is. So *that*, folks, is why flu-like symptoms peak during those months. Most people in this country participating in disruptive eating habits due to traditional festivities are battering their immune systems!

That is also why I never have and probably never will get a flu shot. From the research I have read, it is one of the biggest medical scams around. Don't get me started. My philosophy (which I know is not a popular one) is just eat right and you should never need a shot because chances of you getting the flu are slim.

Note: The recipe for Raw Chocolate Bon-Bons is found on page 79 of *Living Superfood Recipes.*

Now, pardon me while I go lick my fingers.

January 1, 2013

Happy New Year! I am welcoming in this new beginning by thanking God for my health and the health of all my loved ones. I shall honor Him with the first fruits of my harvest.

Speaking of fruit, we purchase lots of it each week from the market. The logic is if it's handy and right there in front of you, you'll begin eating it more often. It can be so *in*expensive as well. We shop at our local Mexican markets where produce is almost half the price of that in major chains. The fruit and veggies are really no different since we don't buy organic produce in a chain grocery store anyway. As long as you wash the items very well, it's all good. Some people prefer to buy bottled vegetable wash, but that's not really necessary. A water and white vinegar combination will work just fine (3:1 ratio). We don't do either. We simply soak our produce in dish detergent (plant-based Seventh Generation works well) and rinse thoroughly.

A typical shopping trip to the Mexican mart has us out the door with about seven bags of fruits and veggies for just $22! That's crazy good! We don't even go to any other section of this store, as there is nothing else there that we would consume.

Today, in addition to our regular items, we got a whole crate of peaches for only $4! It was filled to the brim. They were going to throw them away because they were bruised. Stores also toss out brown spotted bananas, when that's when they are at their peak in nutrition. What? That is our crazy backwards way of operating in this country.

Since there is nothing wrong with bruised fruit when juicing it, we talked to the produce manager and asked him to cut us a deal for the whole bushel. He obliged and that's how we got it so cheap! We had peach nectar for days, as well as peach smoothies, peach yogurt, peach cheesecake. Felt a little "Bubba shrimp" thing going on, but it was all raw, all delicious!

January 6, 2013

We invited a couple of brand-new friends over for dinner, whom we met at a Kwanzaa celebration. During this meal, my daughter, home from college for winter break, finally began to embrace this type of eating. She had been rather hesitant to try any of it prior to this. At first, I thought she became less resistant when seeing how much other people embraced it, as the guests kept going back for more. Then I realized it was simply her discovery of the delicious taste of the highly seasoned, living Superfood meals that got her hooked!

Our meal consisted of spinach-save-my-life soup, living hummus, color garden salad with honey mustard dressing, zucchini wraps, broccoli-cauliflower-ginger salad, avocado-tomato salad, apple sauce, spicy zucchini cheese, and cut vegetables. Barley tea.[19]

February 1, 2013

Mom is visiting. Tonight, she had her first super duper living Superfood feast! She enjoyed it and is attempting to add plant-based foods to her standard diet. Like so many people (me included), the tough part in the beginning stages of eating this way is staying motivated to prepare the meals.

When you're not equipped with all the right appliances (juicer, blender, food processor, dehydrator, etc.) or not around other people eating this way, it does require a little more effort to push through until eating this way becomes a habit.

Like any new business venture, it will require patience. It will all come together eventually, so do not give up! Your organs, your bones, your blood, your joints, and all the systems within your body will love you for pushing through that tough beginning!

Our meal consisted of Essene bread (made in the dehydrator), un-tuna with tomato and alfalfa sprouts, tomato-flax-broccoli crackers, zucchini cheese, yam chips, salsa with blue corn chips, olive-mushroom paté, and zucchini pasta with herb sauce.[20]

Also pictured below is the Excalibur food dehydrator I highly recommend. You can process seven trays of food at one time. Do not mess around with the cheaper plastic models like I did at first. They don't last and are not spacious enough to allow mass production.

February 2, 2013

What did I have for breakfast today? Just a little bit of fruit with a topping that made it oh so tasty but more importantly rewarding for my organs.

This dish consisted of Papaya, kiwi, almond yogurt (made with banana, chia seeds & maple syrup), goji berries, coconut flakes, chocolate powder, cinnamon and garnished with mint leaves.

It was so easy! Who knew just adding little toppings to fruit can change it from a somewhat boring snack to a vitamin-dense, hyper-nutritional meal!

---

[19] Appendix B. page 100. Figure 5.
[20] Appendix B. page 100. Figure 6.

Come on, you can make something tasty like this for your breakfast, right?

Feb 21, 2013

Dinner was delicious! I had Shirataki noodles, aka yam noodles. Whenever we do have cooked noodles (heated in the dehydrator on a very low setting) they are either the yam or Kelp ones; a great substitute for pasta and a healthy one at that. For instance, kelp has a high concentration of iodine, which is important for the thyroid, immune system, and female hormone regulation. Japanese women, who eat a lot of sea kelp are known to have lower rates of ovarian, breast, and endometrial cancer. Sadly, that rate is rising as their diets become more westernized.

You probably don't hear much talk about endometrial cancer. Even though it accounts for only less than one per cent of all cancer deaths, it is the sixth most common cancer in women worldwide. In 2008, around 290,000 new cases were recorded in the U.S., which equaled approximately five percent of all new cases of cancer in women.[21]

The highest rate of endometrial cancer is found in high-income countries, such as North America. Following suit are Central and Eastern Europe, with Middle and Western Africa showing a low rate of incidences.[22] Not giving birth to children adds to the risk.[23]

There is so much to learn about this cancer that tends to strike women more so after menopause. I have not even scratched the surface there, so do your research...and eat some yam or kelp noodles!

My meal consisted of: Shirataki noodles with a "cheesy" non-dairy sauce, jicama "live" fries, cauliflower popcorn, collard salad and cous cous.[24]

---

[21] Ferlay J, Shin HR, Bray F et al. (2008) GLOBOCAN *Cancer Incidence and Mortality Worldwide*: IARC Cancer Base No.10 [Internet]. Lyon, France: International Agency for Research on Cancer; 2010. From globocan.iarc.fr.

[22] Ibid. Page 6.

[23] Ibid. Page 7.

[24] Appendix B. Page 101, Figure 7.

April 13, 2013

Ahhh, a beautiful, sunny Saturday afternoon on the patio at home in front of the newly planted raised bed garden. Even though Chef Keidi started this garden only a month ago, it is already bringing forth food for the table! I picked some kale and dehydrated them into kale chips.[25] They are nicely seasoned and spicy! This is only my second time attempting this. I think I nailed it!

To make kale chips, you marinate the fresh greens for a few minutes in a small amount of olive oil, balsamic vinegar and organic soy sauce. Mix in several seasonings like curry, garlic, turmeric and cayenne pepper. Place the limp leaves on trays in the dehydrator for lots of hours. The time varies depending on how full your dehydrator is; could be 6, 8 or 12 hours. When done, they are spicy, crispy and oh so yummy!

Note: The recipe for Kale/Collards Krisp is found on page 41 of *Superfood Recipes*.

April 27, 2013

My, oh my, I did such a great job making a new recipe called Raw Caramel Slice that I got brave enough to share it with the attendees at our living super food meal demonstration today. They loved it!

This delicious desert consists of: Chocolate (unprocessed), coconut oil and tahini. The crust is made from crushed almonds and dates.[26] It's a rather expensive of a dish to make because of the coconut oil and tahini, but hey, it's worth every penny. Um, mm, good! Remember, it's all uncooked, so it's simple and quick to make. My little chocolate squares didn't turn out exactly like the perfect-looking ones photographed with the recipe I found online, but that's okay. Mine were just as tasty, if not tastier!

---

[25] Appendix B. Page 101, Figure 8.

[26] Appendix B. Page 101, Figure 9.

Note: This recipe can be found on my website, *The Law & Raw Institute for Balanced Healthy Living.* www.law-raw.com/raw-recipes/raw-caramel-slice (I give props to the original source of this recipe on my site.)

May 1, 2013

Lentil burgers[27] prepared in the dehydrator are yummy!

I am still a little intimidated by that whole dehydrating thing. I know I've been around the raw experience long enough I should have it mastered by now. Perhaps I still haven't fully wrapped my brain around the notion of it taking so long for the process to be completed in the dehydrator. Sometimes 12 hours!

You can also use your conventional oven like a dehydrator if you do not own a dehydrator. Simply set the heating temperature between 118 and 125 and leave the door slightly ajar so air can circulate inside. Be prepared, though, to have that oven on for quite a long time.

Years of receiving instant results with our food preparations—thanks to microwave ovens and fast-food restaurants—can create a very impatient person. Be aware, though, the habit of impatience can spill over into a lot of areas of your life, not just in preparing and eating meals.

Note: This recipe for Sprouted Lentil Veggie Burger can be found on page 49 of *Living Superfood Recipes.*

May 2, 2013

Harvest day from our garden! There are so many greens that all look alike to me. I am still learning, so I don't know exactly what all I'm picking. What I do know, though, is that the taste of these greens is so alive and rich in flavor—much more than those purchased from the grocery store!

Who knew we were giving up so much in taste due to all the time it takes transporting the produce from point A to Z. We're also giving up nutrients because of the mass-produced soil not being organic like in one's own backyard.

---

[27] Appendix B. Page 101, Figure 10.

The greens I picked were: Mustard, arugula, fennel, rosemary, thyme, cilantro, basil, marjoram, dill, mint, three types of green lettuce, red chard, spinach, turnip greens, red kale, Russian kale, bok choy, escarole, red romaine and radishes.[28]

Now go to the photo of these beautiful greens and things in the Appendix and see if you can match each of the names listed here to the items there.

May 12, 2013

Happy Mother's Day to me!

My days generally begin in the wee morning hours—the optimal time for my creative writing juices to flow. This morning, a surprise came knocking at my office door: a special Mother's Day breakfast served to me on a tray.

My meal consisted of: Plantain fritters served with maple syrup and homemade strawberry jam, along with mango chunks, hibiscus tea and a sprig of mint from the garden.[29] Um, mm, scrumptious!

As much as I appreciated the delicious cuisine, the thought behind it was cherished even more.

July 15, 2013

Little did I know this raw food journey would open our home to so many dinner guests—old friends and new friends. I love it!

I especially enjoy old friends visiting. So many of them come to Las Vegas for conferences, group outings or vacations and they set aside time to visit me. Those are special visits because there's beautiful synergy when gathering under the auspices of a common past, while partaking of something new and alive.

Most of our dinner guests are tasting this type of food for the very first time. They all come away from the table amazed and loving the food. I knew they would.

---

[28] Appendix B. Page 101, Figure 11.
[29] Appendix B. Page 101, Figure 12.

When these visitors return home, perhaps they will tell all their friends and family about how this delicious raw food really is God's medicine. After all, not *everything* that happens in Vegas should stay here.

Spread the rawsomeness of raw cuisine!

For the serious-minded ONLY, if that's not you, then please skip.

If you are sick and tired of being sick and tired, let's journey together to the land of wellness, free from the confines of America's dangerous and broken health care system. Purchase one of my health-related books, join my 30-day wellness challenge, and also opt for a one-on-one consultation to receive a customized game plan to becoming your healthiest you! Contact me via TerriLiggins.com and let's chat!

Part IV

My Appreciation

In Appreciation

I am grateful for the sense of purpose I have been given by God and the wisdom to understand it. Much respect to the balance Mother Nature provides, blessing me with strength and confidence to unleash my gifts for the world to benefit.

My earthly father gives me the *reason* to keep going each day. Much gratitude and love to you, Dad.

My mother instills in me *belief* that I can keep going each day. Much gratitude and love to you, Mom.

My children, Brittany "Skye" Shepard and Steven Shepard, are the *breath* allowing me to wake up each day with both the reason to go forward and the belief that I can. Thank you and I love you both dearly!

Siblings are the first friends, the first rivals, and often the most profound influences that shape who we become, sometimes even more than our parents. So, to Thom, Theresa, Toni, and Tim, thank you for the wonderful job you did in shaping my life. Over the last 50+ years, your lessons taught through love, encouragement, and even our opposition have been truly invaluable. I appreciate all their spouses as well, for their integral role with my sibs over the years. Much love and respect to all of you!

Shout-out to Cheri for being not only a terrific sis-in-law, but my fantastic editor of many years!

Terri Eileen Liggins

Special hugs and love to all my nieces and nephews and their spouses and offspring. This health journey of mine is for your generation, and those after you, to observe, copy and live it. Please, please, please turn around this atrocious death-by-food crisis the baby boomer generation has allowed to implode.

I've also been blessed with scores of people who have enriched my life— extended family, lifelong friends, sorority sisters, co-workers, and so many others. Although some are no longer physically present, their impact endures, and their memory will always live on in my heart. All have been the much-needed kaleidoscope to this otherwise dull and over-analyzed life of mine. Love and blessings to all of you!

Lastly, thank you, Keidi Obi Awadu, aka Chef Keidi. You are my truest health hero! I'm grateful for our timely reconnection after 50 years. May our partnership in nutritional healing continue to bless multitudes with restored vitality, energy, and longevity along this extraordinary journey called life. Peace and peas to you!

Amen. Asé. Ire.

Part V

APPENDICES

Appendix A
My Diagnoses

My diagnosis of a myocardial infarction (heart attack) in November 1999, along with a second episode in May 2000. My diagnosis of sarcoidosis in June 2000.

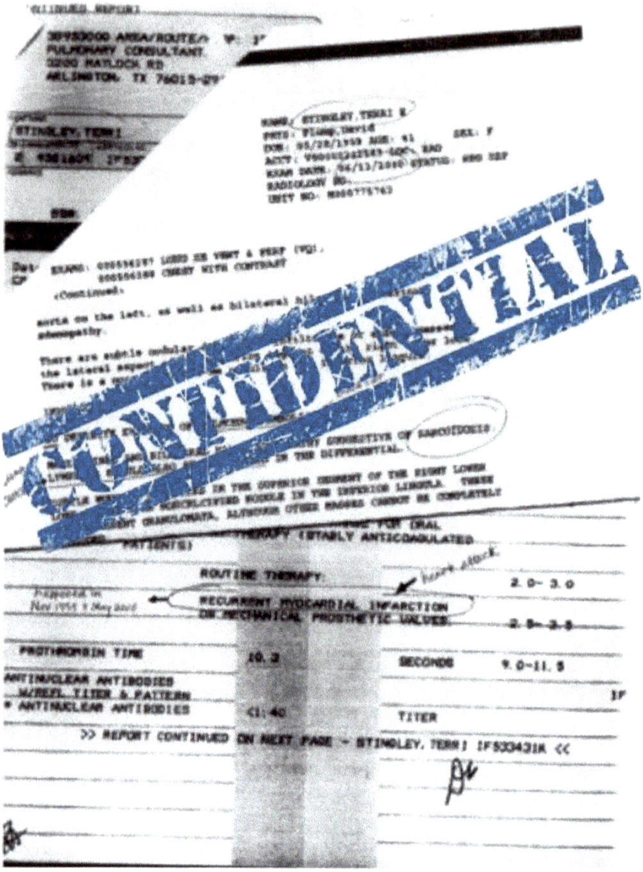

Figure 1

In 2010. The aspiration of breast mass procedure to test for breast cancer upon the discovery of a lump during a mammogram. Findings were benign.

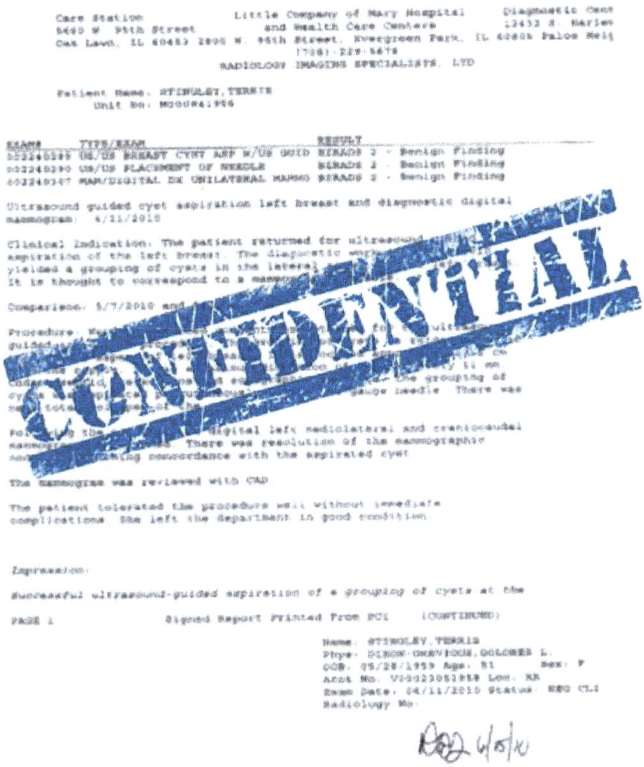

Care Station — Little Company of Mary Hospital and Health Care Centers — Diagnostic Cent

95th Street, Oak Lawn, IL — 95th Street, Evergreen Park, IL — Palos Heig

RADIOLOGY IMAGING SPECIALISTS, LTD

EXAM#	TYPE/EXAM	RESULT
	US/US BREAST CYST ASP W/US GUID	BIRADS 2 - Benign Finding
	US/US PLACEMENT OF NEEDLE	BIRADS 2 - Benign Finding
	MAM/DIGITAL DX UNILATERAL MAMMO	BIRADS 2 - Benign Finding

Ultrasound guided cyst aspiration left breast and diagnostic digital mammogram: 6/11/2010

Clinical Indication: The patient returned for ultrasound guided aspiration of the left breast. The diagnostic work ... yielded a grouping of cysts in the lateral ... It is thought to correspond to a mammo...

Comparison: 5/7/2010 and ...

The mammogram was reviewed with CAD.

The patient tolerated the procedure well without immediate complications. She left the department in good condition.

Impression:

Successful ultrasound-guided aspiration of a grouping of cysts at the

PAGE 1 Signed Report Printed From PCI (CONTINUED)

Figure 2

Appendix B
Photos of Stuff I Eat

Pictured below are actual meals I eat.

Mmm, mmm! They are nutrient-dense meals, which makes them not just raw, but live, super foods—and yummy to boot!

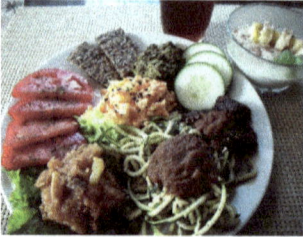

Figure 1. See page 77

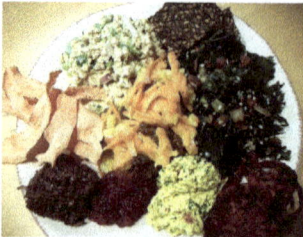

Figure 2. See page 79

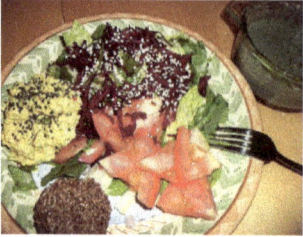

Figure 3. See page 79

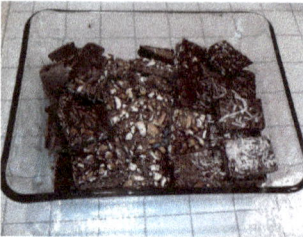

Figure 4. See page 79

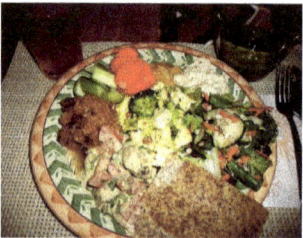

Figure 5. See page 82

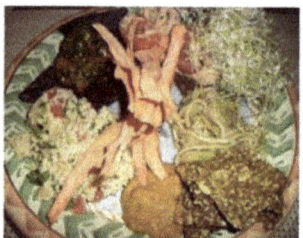

Figure 6. See page 82

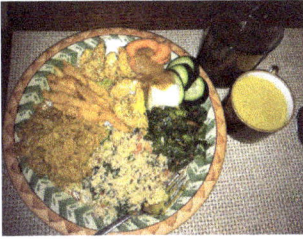

Figure 7. See page 83

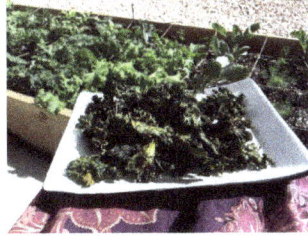

Figure 8. See page 84

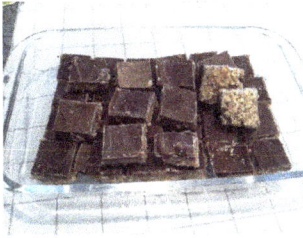

Figure 9. See page 84

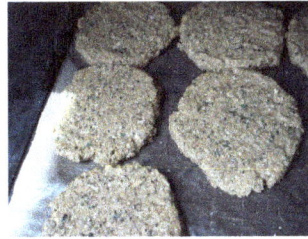

Figure 10. See page 85

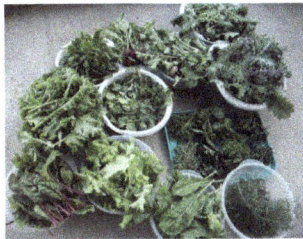

Figure 11. See page 86

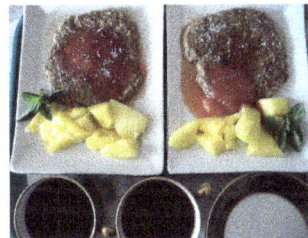

Figure 12. See page 86

Appendix C
My first year completed!

August 22, 2013

Today is my one-year anniversary of going RAW! Yea!

One year of turning back my body's biological clock. One year of ridding my body of serious health challenges. One year of "offing" almost 30 lbs effortlessly. (During the past five years, I've put about 10 pounds back on to the 119 pounds.) One year of learning to love the kitchen (well, let's not push it... learning to LIKE the kitchen). One year of staying on this path to optimum health, wealth and longevity through the consumption of plant-based, hyper-nutrition, live-enzyme foods.

I am **R**eaching **A**nd **W**inning this marathon race called life—staying on course until my ripe age of 120, or until my ENTIRE purpose here on earth has been fulfilled. Here's to whichever one comes first!

Here's to a full spectrum of great tasting, live, super-nutritional foods as the medicine that will help me get there vibrantly and dazzlingly!

Here's to YOUR transition to a healthier YOU, as well! Asé

These first two photos are of me wearing the capris pants I spoke of in Chapter 1. Photo 1: Before going raw. Photo 2: After going raw. Photo 3: Three years after going raw, the weight has stayed off. The weight is still off five years later. Proof that this has been a lifestyle change, not yo-yo dieting.

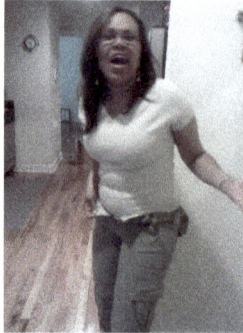

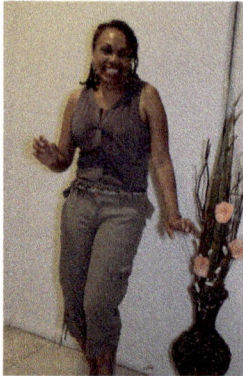

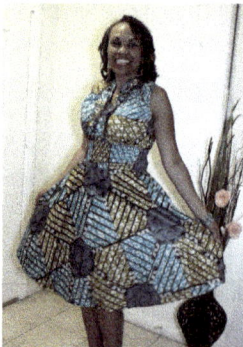

Appendix D
Resources

This book was published by The Literary Front Publishing Company, a firm founded on the belief that every powerful story deserves to be heard. We specialize in ghostwriting for a diverse clientele, from influential public figures to everyday individuals. We are proud to help people with extraordinary victories share their unique stories with the world. www.TheLiteraryFront.com

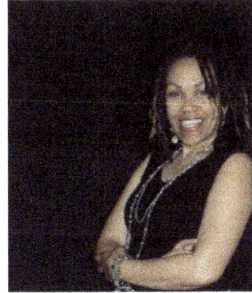

Chef Keidi Awadu is an award-winning raw food chef, researcher and nutritional expert. As a longtime radio journalist, he regularly broadcasts and publishes cutting edge news about societal issues including nutrition, detoxification, disease prevention and longevity. To purchase his Living Superfood series of books, as well other titles from his repertoire of 40+ books, go to www.LivingSuperfood.com.

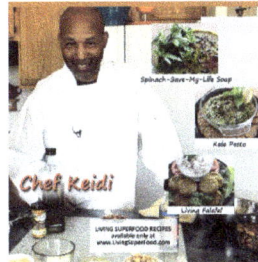

About the Author

Terri Liggins' life changed dramatically at 40 when a mild heart attack and serious autoimmune disease ended her corporate career. In 2000, she turned her passion for writing into purpose, launching a ghostwriting business, bringing extraordinary stories to life for clients including a world-renowned motivational speaker, Les Brown, an international model, retired U.S. Senator, Roland Burris, and top Cleveland Clinic surgeons.

After 12 years of pain, Terri reversed her condition through a 100% raw, plant-based, high-protein lifestyle—becoming symptom-free of all ailments in just seven days! As an unexpected bonus, she dropped 30 pounds over several months. She remains disease-free and shares this healing path through best-selling books, food prep demos, and wellness programs.

Holding advanced degrees in Business and Law, Terri created the **4th Quarter Lifestyle (4QL)** brand, featuring a digital directory and mobile app for baby boomers, caregivers, and forward thinkers, offering education and legacy-building tools like living wills, trusts, and final expenses planning.

This dedicated Boomerpreneur is based in Las Vegas. In her spare time, she loves planning her next exotic journaling retreat, visiting her two children in California, her family in Ohio.

Visit **TerriLiggins.com**.

Additional books by this author:

Fix Your Immune System – With an Anti-Inflammatory Lifestyle

Fix Your Gut – and Get Relief from Celiac, Crohn's, IBD, IBS, GERD, and More

Grateful Me – My Gratitude Journal

My Spiritual Guide to Walking in Excellence – A Psalm 119 Journal

More to come…

For more information on these and future publications, as well as to purchase, go to www.TerriLiggins.com

www.ingramcontent.com/pod-product-compliance
Lightning Source LLC
Chambersburg PA
CBHW071136280326
41935CB00010B/1251